HE CAME IN WITH IT

TURNER PUBLISHING COMPANY

Nashville, Tennessee

www.turnerpublishing.com

HE CAME IN WITH IT

Cover design: Lauren Peters-Collaer

Cover Art: Nick O'Rourke

Book design: Karen Sheets de Gracia

LIBRARY OF CONGRESS CATALOGING-IN-PUBLICATION DATA

Names: Feldman, Miriam, author.

Title: He came in with it : a portrait of motherhood and madness / by Miriam Feldman.

Description: Nashville, Tennessee : Turner Publishing Company, [2020] | Summary: "He Came In With It is the chronology of a mother and her family's coping with mental illness: the hurdles of diagnosis and treatment— of stigma, denial, shame—of pretending that things are T-square perfect for all the lacquered world" —Provided by publisher.

Identifiers: LCCN 2019035587 (print) | LCCN 2019035588 (ebook) | ISBN 9781684425112 (hardback) | ISBN 9781684425129 (paperback) | ISBN 9781684425136 (ebook)

Subjects: LCSH: Feldman, Miriam. | Feldman, Miriam—Family. | O'Rourke, Nick (Nicholas Dylan)— Mental health. | Parents of mentally ill children—United States—Biography. | Schizophrenics— United States—Biography. | Schizophrenia in children—United States. | Schizophrenics—Family relationships—United States. | Mothers and sons—United States.

Classification: LCC RJ506.S3 F45 2020 (print) | LCC RJ506.S3 (ebook) | DDC 616.89/80092 [B]—dc23

LC record available at https://lccn.loc.gov/2019035587

LC ebook record available at https://lccn.loc.gov/2019035588

PRINTED IN THE UNITED STATES OF AMERICA

20 21 22 23 24   10 9 8 7 6 5 4 3 2 1

HE CAME IN WITH IT

A PORTRAIT OF MOTHERHOOD AND MADNESS

MIRIAM FELDMAN

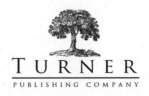

TURNER
PUBLISHING COMPANY

For my mother

In a rock cleft wall
Crumbling, vine covered—
I lean my weary head against the stone
Absorbing the last sun brightness
Half conscious only that the early evening breeze
Has begun
And the trees whisper and sigh.

The bird and the cricket noises
And the tree lizards, too, I think,
Come tumbling in the breech the wind has opened
Crowding back my jumbled thoughts
So I must forsake them for a moment
To look
And smell and hear the world,

The hills have changed.
I fell into my reverie
When they were brown, red and green and ochre
With occasional patches of burnt scrub
And now they've changed to purple nubby silhouettes,
The molten sky
Their swiftly changing backdrop.

But at my right
The brilliant blue endured
The trees and grass flame green in golden light.
The breeze is now a steady wind
It drives the clacking leaves along
They skip
And disappear from sight.

Would that such a wind
Cool, with healing gift
Would enter the fissures of my soul
And sweep it clean
Of all the left over, re-warmed odds and ends
Of living
That clutter and stifle it.

Poor soul of mine
Which cannot look out
Through its windows blocked
With useless sentiments.
I promise you a grand spring cleaning
Tomorrow
When I have slept.

The stone is warm
Beneath my burdened head
Perhaps thankfulness for constant things
Like the loveliness of land
And that the sun always sets so new days will come
Would bring
A peace not born of little things.

—Lillian Weiss
February 12, 1949
San Juan Hueyapan, Mexico

1

SON

I guess there were signs. There had to have been signs. I missed them all.

So where does this story begin? Damned if I know, exactly. I had me a son. I had a fat little baby boy with a mouth like a rubber band. My husband, Craig, and I surfed the labor waves together like champs. When my son came out of me, the room was oddly hushed. He was my first, so I didn't know what to expect. But it sure was quiet in there. No slap and cry, no nothing. Nick was blue and cold when he was born. We waited in the delivery room for his inaugural wail and heard only silence.

"Don't worry, dear," the nurse said. "We just have to warm him up a bit."

They placed him in an apparatus that looked like a toaster oven. Everything in the room seemed cold, frozen. My husband and I each held our breath, and finally our son took his first. And we let ours out. I had my boy. Deep dark eyes and a serious composure. All the fingers, all the toes.

We named him Samuel, as we had planned, and then after a day or two, Craig and I renamed him Nicholas. Nick. I'd had a beloved uncle with that name, so that was fine with me. Craig gave him the middle name Dylan, after Bob.

Nick: a normal, healthy boy. He was strong, he was adorable, and his future was as bright as the goddamned sun. I would loll around and stare at that future of his like a baby myself, entranced with jangling keys. Now Nick sits in a dark room all day, each day, and I wonder, what is he thinking? Who is in there?

I see how people look at him. I can read my family's faces. I know what has happened to him is a tragedy. But to me he is in there, and his future is still ablaze, alone in his filthy apartment that I try to keep clean.

It was a soft, white afternoon on Ridgewood Place. Saturdays were generally quiet; an occasional dog would bark, but hours could go by without so much as the sound of a slow-moving car. A pleasant melancholy settled in on the weekends.

Walking a few houses up the street to collect Nick from a play-date with his friend Jack, I felt an overall sense of goodness and well-being. We had managed to buy our first house in Larchmont Village, an idyllic neighborhood of Los Angeles. I was a working artist, I had a handsome husband, and we had a darling son and another baby on the way. We seemed to belong perfectly in this venerable neighborhood where generations of families had deep roots in old homes. All was going as planned.

It had rained. As I walked, the sun came out, throwing long shadows and a crispness into the air. Everything felt fresh. With each step, wet leaves underfoot, the sidewalk felt comfortable. I was on my block. I was in my life.

My neighbor's porch was still dripping. Nick was waiting for me on the steps with Jack and his mother, Bridget. We chatted for a minute, then I took his hand and we began down the sidewalk.

"Did you have fun, Nickboy? Was it a good day?" I asked.

"Yeah, we lined up all the toys, the little ones. They stretched all around the living room."

He loved to do that, make long, domino-like trails of objects winding through the rooms of the house. He also utilized endless quantities of tape to sculpt airplanes and monsters. He made them out of clay sometimes too.

"Well, that sounds good," I said.

"Ma, what's the thing about shadows?" he asked, squinting into the sun.

"The thing?"

"I mean, like right now, my shadow is really long. But it changes all the time. Why?"

We stopped for a minute, and I crouched down. "You know how the earth revolves around the sun, so in the morning the sun rises, moves across the sky, and then sets on the other side?"

"Yes."

"In the morning, our shadows stretch in one direction as the sun moves up and across, so they get longer and longer, like now." I pointed to our lengthy shapes on the cement, stretching into the rich amber light. I stood up, and we continued walking. "Isn't it wonderful, Nicky, the way our shadows are always with us? They're like our best friends. Isn't that a lovely thing?"

My four-year-old looked up at me with his endless brown eyes and smiled. "Yes," he said. "And when we die, we will go into our shadows."

At the time, I marveled at what a profound thought that was. Surely, this was evidence that he was no ordinary child. He was some kind of savant with the soul and vision of an adult. This was a child destined to do important things. And I was a young mother filled with the hubris of inexperience.

Nick and his father were inseparable. From the time Nick was a toddler, Craig took him everywhere. They went on fishing trips and to museums, sharing a private bond. It was an antidote for the pain of neglect Craig had suffered at his own father's hand. Most nights, after dinner, Nick followed Craig out to his studio in the garage.

My husband is an artist. When he works, he sits, formally, at his easel. His paintings are abstracts—clean, geometric composition juxtaposed with rich, painterly technique. They line the white walls of his studio, positioned carefully with tape measures and levels.

"Dad is the opposite of you, Mama," Nick said one evening. "When you paint, it flies all over the place. You even put the brushes in your mouth!"

"Yep, Nickboy, I think your dad could paint in a tuxedo."

Nick was in karate pants, no shirt, maybe seven years old. He lay sprawled on the floor of the neat studio, big torn white butcher paper all around him, his supplies a jumble. He was working on a large tempera painting of a farmyard, with cows and chickens and pigs behind a meticulously rendered fence. He had shaded the animals in a way that showed their shapes and three-dimensionality. The sky wasn't just a simple blue; it was light at the horizon and moved to a deep cobalt at the top.

At open house night, the other parents would whisper to each other in front of his artwork. I knew he was good. In my mind's eye, there was a bright image: Nick spinning the world on the tip of his finger. I stood by, expectantly, waiting to see what marvelous things he would do with his life.

I started writing over ten years ago, when Nick was about twenty. That is where I mark the official beginning of the time I call the Bad Ten Years. It hasn't all been terrible. Some of it has been quite funny. Some of it profound in a way I never knew life could be. Although the decade point is where I roughly place the onset, his decline certainly started long before. I have reimagined every minute of his life, trying to find the foreshadowing I must have missed. Where was the exact moment of portent? And how did I not see it?

Nick did fall off the bed when he was a baby. He did. Onto the floor and onto his head. I cannot deny it. I looked away for a moment, and he rolled right off. There is also the chilling footage—

on VHS tape—of a backyard barbeque at my brother's house. Nick is only a year old. He topples over, and his head smacks down on a stepping-stone. His aunt's and uncle's gasps are audible on the film. Craig is behind the camera. I watch that one repeatedly. In the footage, I pick him up and rock him in my arms.

"You're fine. It's just a little bump," I say.

I sound so confident, so unconcerned. I rub his little head and talk in a soothing voice. There is nothing that Mama's love can't fix. Did that bang on the head cause the schizophrenia? How will I ever know?

For a decade, my mind has been a churning chorus of voices questioning my alacrity, my awareness, my own timing and perceptions. I question everything I have ever done.

I agonized over every morsel I put into my body while I was pregnant with him. I did drink some beer from time to time before I knew I was pregnant. I regularly took melatonin to sleep during the nine months. Did that ruin his brain? Was that it? Or is it heredity? This, I know, plagues my husband terribly. There is some mental illness in his lineage. There is depression too. Craig suffers from it. He is a sixth cousin of Winston Churchill, who is said to have been bipolar. Tiny buds on his family tree emerge and connect to articulate blame. Too often, that guilt and liability insinuate themselves in our marriage.

Or perhaps we were just lousy parents?

Sixty years ago, psychiatrists blamed the mother for schizophrenia. There was an actual term: the refrigerator mother theory. It put forth the notion that the disease was caused by the mother's remoteness and lack of warmth. So along with the searing ache and helplessness, mothers were also asked to shoulder the blame. This has changed, but the medical community still does not know why schizophrenia occurs. Experts agree there is a genetic component, but they cannot separate with any certainty the physiological causes from the environmental ones.

In his early teens, Nick began to bite his nails. They were always ragged and sometimes bloody.

"You've got to break that habit, kiddo. Your hands are a mess."

"I know, Ma," he said. "I'm just kind of nervous a lot."

"Well, find some other way to cope. Maybe jumping jacks?" I always thought I had the simple answer.

Nick discovered that marijuana relaxed him just fine.

I never even asked why he was nervous. I knew about the pot, but I was too distracted to dig any deeper. I carry that guilt on my back now, every day, like a pack mule. Did my desire to present an unblemished veneer cause me to miss the signs? Throw that one up on my shoulders. The rucksack is getting pretty heavy right about now.

I remember, too, a time when I walked by his open bedroom door—he must have been about fifteen then—and saw him lying on his bed after school. I knew he had broken up with his first girlfriend. His face was to the wall, and he covered it with his arm. I sat on his bed, covered with the same bedspread I'd had as a child. My mother had been in the Red Cross during World War II, stationed in Calcutta, India. She'd had the heavy cotton bedsheets block printed in brilliant traditional designs and brought them home to use as bedspreads. Her name, Lillian Weiss, was pressed into the corner of each one. I spent many nights as a child looking at the elephants and dancing women, dreaming of going to India one day myself.

"What's going on, Boychik? You're looking sad."

"Oh, it's the Emily thing, Mom. I feel so bad." He rolled toward me and uncovered his face. He'd been crying.

"I know you feel bad. It's the worst feeling. You probably think this isn't possible, but really, in the scope of your life, this is going to be a little blip. There will be so many more girls. You'll meet that right person, and this won't matter at all." My misguided comment effectively dismissed his pain.

He turned back to the wall. "I'm afraid of my own thoughts, Ma.

You just can't understand what's going on in my head. I have these thoughts that are scary, they're bad, and I don't know what to do about them."

This was not what I wanted to hear. This delivered its own lingering shade filled with serious implications. I wanted to keep things normal.

"Oh, Nick," I said. "Everybody has weird thoughts and crazy ideas. It's nothing to stress about. What matters is what you do, not what you think. There is nothing to feel guilty about." Fine, that sounded good. Let's just add: "What really matters are our actions, Nick, so please don't worry about your thoughts."

Idiot. Please don't worry about your thoughts? Perfect thing to tell a person developing a thought disorder. He was hearing voices!

Was that the onset of everything? Could I have saved him if I had been smarter, more aware? I'd been given a whisper from the future, and I ignored it. If one compiled a list of the red flags for mental illness and then a list of normal teenage behaviors, it might well be the same list: mercurial emotions, inability to focus, inconsistent behavior, lack of interest in school. Nick didn't seem any different from all the rest of the kids. But in my gut, there had been a rumbling. I just hadn't wanted to hear it.

The truth is that I cannot point to where it all started. Our son was slowly erased and replaced by someone else. What can possibly prepare you for that? You fret and suffer, striving to protect your children from the instant you push them out of you. You prepare yourself for the worst things that can happen to them. You think about cancer, envision car accidents, and fear abductions. Who among us is prepared for the disappearance of your child into his own mind?

And suddenly, in the loop of memories that plays on and on in my head, I am careening back to an earlier time. When Nick was five, he asked me about death.

"What happens when you die?"

Oh, I was ready for that one. "Sit down, Nicky, and we can talk about it."

I laid it out. I talked about our spirits. I discussed, on his level, the inevitability of dying. As I listened to my own wisdom waft through the air, I thought, *Oh my God, I am a great mother.*

I explained the interconnectedness of all life forces, skimmed lightly over the charming idea of heaven, discussed various religions and their approaches to the subject. I thought, *Look at him. Look at him! He is in rapt attention, understanding every word! He is staring directly at my mouth, that's how fascinated he is.*

When I had finished my polished and penetrating explanation of death, I gazed lovingly at Nick and asked, "Do you have any questions?"

"What's inside your lips?"

I suppose I should have known then that I did not have this mother thing down. But that was a long time ago, before things fell apart in a way I never could have anticipated. When it happened, there was only one fact: I had lost my son. Not in the way that one misplaces something, not lost as in death, but lost to me in a way that blindsided me. Lost to me in bits and pieces over time, like falling leaves. Lost to me in a way I didn't comprehend and hated with a virulence that could level the world. Nick was in front of me, all in one piece, not conspicuously torn, still recognizable. All there and yet not Nick anymore. Not my son.

2

IT BEGINS

Nick at sixteen had been spending most weekends at a friend's house in Topanga Canyon with a group of pals. My husband was not too keen on this; he suspected all kinds of bad behavior. But as was typical in my all-too-frequent episodes of "I know best," I outlasted him and what I dismissed as his negativity. I had it all under control. Our rule for Nick was that he had to call from a landline upon his arrival and check in throughout the weekend. Everything under control. Of course, in actuality, he was gallivanting all over doing terrible drugs that probably exacerbated the as yet undiagnosed schizophrenia. But I had imposed a rule for checking in, so all was well.

It was very early on a Sunday morning, and we were all sleeping. The phone rang at 4:45 a.m.

I'd drilled into my kids' heads that they could call me anytime if they were in trouble. No questions asked, I would come get them. I was informed by a recording that I had a collect call.

"Ma, could you come pick me up?" Nick said in a rasp.

"What happened? Where are you? What's wrong?"

"I just need you to come get me."

It was still dark when I left the house. Los Angeles is a big, full city, but at certain times it shimmers like an empty stage set, waiting for the show to start. I drove through that vacuum in a state of suspended animation, trying to make out shapes.

As I think back now to that morning, I want to grab on to the previous day and never let go. The funny thing is, I can't for the life of me even remember what we did on Saturday. Our last day before the storm. Did I do chores and drive the girls around? Did Craig and I go out together? Was I in a bad mood, wasting the last clean, carefree day of my life?

The light had started to rise, a thin blue black, as I pulled to the curb where Nick stood. It was too dark to see that he didn't have his backpack. Too dark to see that he had lost his phone. No way to know that he was emerging from a furious drug odyssey that had wrung out his brain. But I *could* make out that he was covered in grass, leaves, and dirt.

"What the hell did you do, Nick, crawl through the bushes?" I barked.

Not the most palliative salutation considering the circumstances.

He sat beside me in the car and mumbled answers to my barrage of questions. He had been with friends, and they all did mushrooms. He'd left his companions, lost his cell somewhere between the house and the roadside. Left his backpack . . . somewhere . . . and wandered around for a while. Finally, he had summoned the fortitude to find a phone and call me.

It was one of those lost mornings. The move from night to day was impossible to gauge, wondrous and vague. A big gray sky slipped across the city, pushing aside the darkness, leaving the moon behind. The sun, a wraith, hung nearby. It was difficult to decide who was the intruder—each half of the dim couple seemed to belong. My son was slumped against the door with his arm over his eyes.

The sun broke through, and it was officially day. I took in the sad portrait next to me, and something jumped out that I hadn't noticed before: his arm was covered in blood.

"What in God's name is going on, Nick?" I wailed in my banshee voice. "What is all that blood?"

There were several jagged, messy wounds on his right wrist. I pulled the car to the side of the road. We sat there. In one blinding moment, everything changed. Something very, very bad was happening. There was no more pretending. All the missed signals and clues from which I had turned away were illuminated now. They were written in red on the soft part of his inner arm.

"Let me see."

He listlessly held out his arm. It wasn't actively bleeding.

"Did you do this to yourself?"

"Yeah," he muttered.

"Why?" I looked at him, lost. "Why?"

He gradually told me the rest of the story: Having taken too many—*too many?*—mushrooms, he'd run out of the house into the night and, scared by what his mind was doing, had curled up in some shrubbery and cried. Then he took his Boy Scout pocketknife out and started attacking his wrist.

"Why would you do that? Did you want to die? Were you trying to die?"

"I don't know," he said flatly. "I don't think so."

The lighter it got, the less I could see. The road behind me was a mess, scattered with abandoned items. Close by, somewhere, I imagined Nick's backpack, his knife, his favorite sweatshirt. A little farther back lay my belief that he was just having normal teenage problems. Farther back behind his sweatshirt lay a sunny stretch of highway, with a Boy Scout troop camping in the field nearby. Nick is ten, the image of tousled boyhood, the glint of a blade as he whittles a branch. Way, *way* back there, maybe before the road had even been paved, was my baby boy spinning a globe on his index finger. That's where I wanted to be.

But I wasn't there. I was in the car with my bleeding son, and like in the delivery room on the day he was born, I didn't know what was going on. I turned and looked straight at him. "We are going to figure this out, Nick," I said firmly, confidently. But I was scared to death.

We have three girls and a boy. I've always loved that configuration. Nick was the adored man-child in a world of girls. Our oldest, Scarlett, is Craig's daughter from a brief earlier marriage. She is ten years older than Nick, a sufficient gap of years that effectively separates her from the real-time chaos at home. She was already married when his illness emerged. Lucy is three years younger than Nick, and Rose is three years younger than Lucy. When Nick became ill, Lucy was thirteen and idolized her brother. He had opened her world up to art and music, and she devoured every bit. Rose, an adoring nine-year-old who could always make her brother laugh, was happy just to be near him.

When Rose was about two years old, we went to a pool party at a friend's home. They had hired a lifeguard so the adults could relax. I was talking to some friends when, out of the corner of my eye, I saw some commotion stirring by the Jacuzzi. Our friend Bing Jackman was stepping out of the water and had Rose in his arms. Even from a distance I could see that she was a funny color.

I bolted across the grass. Once I got up close, I saw that her lips were blue. I grabbed her from Bing, lay her over my shoulder, and instinctively started pounding her on the back with an open palm. She didn't move. People gathered around, seemingly in slow motion, with no voices. I continued, calm and focused. Finally, Rose opened her mouth and out gushed a fountain of water that did not seem to subside. It was shocking, more water than one could ever imagine coming out of a little body like hers. She coughed, pinked up, and eventually looked at me and smiled. She settled into my arms and slept, and I held her, watching her, until she awoke an hour later.

Sitting by the pool, holding my two-year-old, I imagined what had happened. The first thing they say a small child does is inhale a deep breath of water. I saw her opening her eyes, submerged, thinking, *Where is my mother?*

"Oh my God, Bing. She would have drowned if it weren't for you. What happened?"

"Mimi, I know that it sounds crazy, but I was lounging there by myself, and as I drifted, it was like someone was saying *open your eyes*. It was spooky, almost like a whisper. Or someone tapping me lightly on the shoulder. I looked up and saw something at the bottom of the Jacuzzi. It was Rose. I just reached down and picked her up, and then you were there. I didn't do anything really, just opened my eyes at the right time."

For months afterward I lay awake, night after night, reliving that day. How could I have let my guard down? How could I have trusted someone else to watch my child? At my core I believe that ultimately the mother is the responsible party, and I couldn't forgive myself.

Opened his eyes at the right time. Tell me, who whispered to Bing Jackman? Who made him look down at precisely the most crucial and urgent moment, in order that he might save Rose? I would like to locate that being. Where has this vigilant inchoate lifeguard gone, now that Nick is slowly drowning in crazy?

When Rose was about five, I asked her if she remembered being at the bottom of the Jacuzzi. She said that she did. I asked her if she was scared. She said no.

"I was safe, Mom. I knew you'd get me."

She remembered feeling safe deep under the warm water. Looking at Nick that Sunday morning in the car, I wondered if he, too, could possibly feel safe under the weight of all his water. I doubted it.

I bought lots of fresh new bandages and first-aid supplies and tended to his arm in the car on the way home.

"Why does Nick have all those Band-Aids on his arm?" Rose asked as we walked in.

Nick silently went upstairs.

"He hurt himself, but he'll be fine."

As we talked behind closed doors, I stressed to Craig that we shouldn't tell the younger girls. It would be too upsetting at their ages. We did tell Scarlett, who now lived in Oregon with her husband and new baby.

I didn't talk about it to my brother, Danny, who lived about a half hour away with his own growing family. In those days, I was still luxuriating in the privileged waters of pointless activity like sibling rivalry. My sister, Sara, lived nearby with her son, who was a bit younger than Nick. We had always been competitive. I wanted to look like I had the better kids, I was the best mom, and other things that have no relevance whatsoever once you enter Crazytown. I detested being vulnerable and did not open up even to close friends. I didn't know then that the constellation of women in my life was what would save me, over and over again.

"He's just lazy," Craig would state with certainty. "That's all that's wrong with him."

Well, he'd been right about the weekends in Topanga Canyon. But no, that couldn't be all there was to it. I'd heave one of my long-suffering sighs. "There is something else going on here. He's sick. We need to help him."

"Oh, right, he's sick. He's 'crazy.' He's crazy like a fox! Maybe if you'd stop wiping up after him, he'd buck up and get it together."

There was definitely some truth in that, but I wasn't ready to see it. I have also learned in the many years since that this is a typical reaction from fathers. They see their sons as versions of themselves and interpret the markers of mental illness as signs of weakness, failure. He was seeing in Nick parts of himself that terrified him.

We are both painters, Craig and I; that is the framework of our marriage. My paintings are realistic depictions of people interacting with the natural world. I love explosions and rough weather. Volcanos. Tornados. I show my work in a gallery. I also run a successful decorative painting business. I paint murals and designs in the big houses and swanky businesses of LA. A lot of my artist friends regard that as a compromise, a sellout, but I get to paint every day of my life, so it's fine with me. Craig is a solitary painter, quietly exploring the liminal world between lines and shapes, earning his living as a woodworker.

We honor each other's primary engagement of lives devoted to making art. It had always held us together when other differences arose. But as our son descended into madness and we followed, we were pulled to a place that threatened all we had built.

As things escalated, I started hiding the events that I thought too frightening to share with the girls. I also stopped telling Craig about Nick's destruction of property at the house. I spackled holes punched in walls, I threw away broken dishes—incriminating evidence that would show I wasn't in control. I presented an edited version of what was going on, because I thought I could handle everything better alone.

After Nick cut his wrist, Craig and I agreed that he would be on lockdown indefinitely. One night he was climbing the walls, pacing all around his room.

"Mom, can't I just go meet Jenny for a coffee?" He was breathing unevenly. His eyes were bright.

I was terrified all the time. I was no longer able to be a good mother, to make good decisions, because I was always in fight-or-flight mode, just trying to keep things from blowing up. Strategies evaporated; promises to my husband to be tougher just melted away.

"No. Definitely not. You know the rules." Even at that point I knew I was going to cave. He looked like he might combust. A thin sheen of sweat shone on his forehead, and he was flicking the forefinger and thumb on his left hand frantically.

"You don't understand—I'm freaking out. I just need some air. I don't know what I'm going to do." We both looked at his wrist.

And there it was, the thing that terrified me most. I *didn't* know what he might do, and giving in seemed like the only way to reduce the risk of him harming himself. I let him go see Jenny. When Craig learned, he was furious.

"I cannot believe you let him go, Miriam. We agreed on this. You never back me up!"

When Nick got back from seeing Jenny, he and Craig had the predictable confrontation in the dining room. After Craig rebuked him, Nick pushed him in the chest. Craig stumbled backward, knocking a picture off the wall. From there, it devolved into a terrible, violent fight, with hitting and furniture flying. Father and son circling each other in battle. Father hitting mother as she intervenes. Mother screaming for them to stop. All of this in front of the girls. To this day I feel sick when I think of that night. I know I shouldn't have let Nick go without talking to Craig, and doing so ignited a fire I couldn't control.

Rose and Lucy did exactly what they saw people do on TV: they called 911. I was mortified. Nick, Craig, and I were still screaming when the girls told us they had called. Immediately I tried to undo what had been done. I grabbed the phone and hit redial.

"Hi, hello, this is Mrs. O'Rourke, my daughters just called you. Everything is fine over here," I said, trying to laugh. "It's all just a terrible misunderstanding. It's all over now. Everything is fine."

I was politely informed that once a call for domestic violence had been made, the police were required to investigate. I scurried around, cleaning the place up, righting furniture and concealing breakage under layers of kitchen garbage. Suddenly, there were helicopters overhead, bright lights, pounding on the door.

Well, this won't draw any attention from the neighbors, I thought, still with one foot in the world where my serene home was intact. I am sure I barely even noticed Rose and Lucy, sitting in the kitchen, crying. Lucy was whispering fervently to her little sister. Rose had a puffy face with snot dripping everywhere.

I put on my well-practiced Everything-Is-Fine mask, walked purposefully to our front door, and opened it, inviting the world of police, paramedics, psych wards, and seventy-two-hour holds into my beautiful Craftsman home.

The cops came in, one woman and two men. They were nice. I had no complaints about them, but I wanted to exit my own life immediately. They took the girls aside separately to ask for their versions of the events. I stood in my dining room, in my nice house on my nice street, and witnessed the slow-motion dissolution of everything I had thought was solid. The shattered glass hidden quickly in the trash can. The broken side chair thrown into the hall closet. Images of family violence seared permanently into Lucy's and Rose's brains.

When they were satisfied there was no imminent danger, and after taking statements from each member of the household, the police left.

The girls went up to bed after being assured by us, repeatedly, that they had done nothing wrong. Then I told Craig he had to leave, the violence was unacceptable. His anger and my betrayal were too much for us as a couple that night. The house could not contain the combined pressure of our conflict, the girls' fear, and all the crazy. The thing is, even then I thought I was okay. I still believed I could handle it—handle Nick—if everyone would just give me complete control. I sat in our bedroom and watched the way Craig's headlights moved across the trees as he left.

Years later, the teenaged Rose hurled the pent-up accusation at me: "The police came to our house, Dad left, and the next day you acted like nothing had happened. You never even mentioned it again!" She was not wrong.

I crumpled at the density of those words. What had all my posing and playacting done to her? What had it done to our relationship? What had it done to her opinion of me?

And so, we return to the pools. The pool Rose almost drowned in. The one full of unimportant concerns in which I could no longer afford to float. The ominous liquid world into which Nick was dissolving. The cold, lonely one in which I now see my husband swam.

I just wanted an army of Bing Jackmans to come save us all.

What followed that awful night were days, nights, years where we just floundered about, trying to figure out what was happening. We were still far from calling it mental illness—that was another world where other people lived. Here, in lovely Larchmont Village, we simply had a troubled kid.

We found a therapist for Nick. That therapist determined after six sessions that his suicide attempt was in fact "inauthentic," which allowed me to delude myself further. I watched the wound, fading under cocoa butter and time, change to a scar and let myself believe "it" was over. For a while, we thought we were dealing with drug abuse. That was a concept I could understand. We flopped in and out of doctors' offices and outpatient rehab programs. The diagnoses kept changing, overlapping—depression, anxiety, addiction—making it impossible, I now see, for us to adhere to a single consistent and sustained approach. It was a moving target.

Meanwhile, in a kind of "for Nick's sake" truce, Craig and I agreed on the notion that we simply had to love him enough; we just hadn't found the right therapist yet; he only needed to stop doing drugs.

But we disagreed on almost everything foundational in day-to-day management of the family. He wanted to be tougher, to discipline "it" out of him. I kept hoping "it" would go away.

The period of time that haunts me most now is his teenage years, when he wasn't yet eighteen and we still had control over his treatment. What if we had gotten him on medication earlier? What if I hadn't been such a fool about his drug usage? We could have put him in a rehab facility. He might have detoxed and never gotten sick at all. We would have been able to understand the indications of his behavior and minimized risk. The fomenting schizophrenia might never have materialized. On my back, staring at the ceiling, these questions consume me night after night.

One morning I received a call from the monsignor at the church around the corner. *What in the world could this be?* Craig attended St. Brendan's, but I am Jewish. We never went to either the church or temple as a family. It turned out, however, that Nick had just paid a visit to the priest at the crack of dawn. We hadn't even known he'd been out of bed.

"I don't want to upset you, Mrs. O'Rourke, but I felt compelled to let you know about my conversation with Nick," the monsignor said kindly. "He wanted to talk about God and things of a spiritual nature. This is not uncommon for young people of his age. But I have counseled many over the years, and there were some troubling aspects to your son's questions. His sense of reality seemed to be a little awry."

"Was there anything in particular?" I asked, wishing I didn't have to.

"No, not really. He asked about heaven and hell and redemption. After all these years, I have a second sense about these things. Keep an eye on him, Mrs. O'Rourke. If there is anything we at the church can do, please do not hesitate to reach out."

There was no disagreement between Craig and me this time. This was disturbing. We asked Nick about it. We approached the subject tenderly and in rare togetherness—that alone was a new dynamic for Nick to experience from his parents—and he dismissed his initiation of that visit as "no big deal." He'd just been walking by the church and decided to amble in. At 5:00 a.m. He gave us one of those obsequious looks a driver might give a cop who had pulled him over. Then he went upstairs.

Nick managed to finish his last semester of high school by doing a home study program. He began community college. He lived at home, a place that had become pretty unbearable for all of us. Nick and Craig were in constant conflict. Craig and I were building resentments and grudges that would take years to resolve. Nick was inappropriate and disruptive with the girls.

"Lucy, your clothes are pretty sexy. You're going to make all the boys horny."

"Mom! Tell him to shut up. That's gross."

"Nick, just go upstairs. Lucy, ignore him. He's just trying to get your goat."

We had always been tough when it came to chores. From the time the kids were little, they were responsible for making their beds and keeping their rooms clean. Overall household chores were added as they got older—dishes, laundry, yard work. Nick's job was to clean up the backyard after the family dog, Buster, daily.

"Nick, there is dog crap all over the yard," Craig would announce daily, and the arguing commenced. Consequences were unenforceable. I would cringe in the house while they fought. I began secretly picking up the goddamned dog shit myself. I just wanted the yelling to stop.

In order to prove his commitment to being clean, Nick decided to quit smoking. He swore he wasn't doing drugs. But we were not born yesterday, so we tested him. One day I was at our neighborhood Rite Aid, just picking up the usual supplies, like all the moms: nicotine patches, urine test kits, Visine, a huge bottle of Rolaids with an extra one hundred tablets, and an even larger bottle of Aleve. I threw all this stuff onto the counter and met the gaze of our dear Muhammad, who worked the cash register. I imagine they train cashiers to not react to or comment about the items purchased. But this was just such a distressing pile of sundries that it was impossible not to bear witness aloud.

"Welcome to my life," I said. We exchanged solemn little smiles, and I left.

Years later we found out from Lucy that Nick had been paying his baby sister—whose adoration had no limits—to pee in a bottle, which he surreptitiously transferred into the drug test container while Dad was standing guard with his back turned. Because, like I said, we weren't born yesterday.

Nick overslept constantly. He went out at night. He dropped classes. This was a sharp change from the boy we had known. He used to work hard, get good grades, and do all kinds of extracurricular activities. He'd held a job at a trendy store on Larchmont. He was a Boy Scout, for God's sake. When all his friends had dropped out because it wasn't cool anymore, he'd stayed, setting his sights on the coveted Eagle Scout rank. "It will help me get into a good college," he'd told me confidently. Now I had to wake him up and give him pep talks just to get him out of the house to community college.

"Nick, I understand this had been a hard time," I said one morning, "but hiding under the covers is not going to make it any better. You have to deal with your problems and get your life back on track."

"I want to, Mom, I really do."

"So do it! Nick, you've always been such a good student. All you need to do is buckle down and finish this year, and then you can go to art school."

"That's what I want to do. I just keep messing up." He looked at me sadly.

"It's your choice whether you mess up or not. You simply have to decide to do the right thing. This is your life, Boyo."

"Something is different, Mom. Back in high school I was the smartest kid. I always had great ideas. Now I don't know anymore."

"What do you mean? You're as smart as you ever were. You're just rusty. You've been messing around for too long. You'll catch up."

"It's not that, Ma. It's something else. When I do participate, when I do talk about my ideas, people look at me like I'm weird. I feel like they don't understand what I'm saying."

"I'm sure you're imagining that. If you were prepared and did the work, you'd be fine." I was still, somehow, operating from my default mothering setting—the one that applies to normal kids.

Now when I recall that discussion, a chill goes down my spine. Of course. Of course they were looking at him like he was weird. He was beginning to have disorganized thoughts, one of the markers for schizophrenia. He probably *didn't* make sense. In a few months, his father and I would be looking at him the same way.

When he was twelve, I signed Nick up for Cotillion at the Wilshire Ebell Theatre, a hundred-year-old social club. Cotillion was supposed to teach the budding young boys and girls good manners; it was very old-fashioned. Craig took him to the men's shop on Larchmont and bought him his first suit. All he needed was shoes.

I had a pair of Doc Martens that would fit him. I didn't see why he couldn't just wear them rather than spend a bunch of money on a new pair.

As we drove to Cotillion, he pouted, gleaming eyes, flushed cheeks. "This really sucks," he said.

"What?"

"Well, I'm pretty sure I'm going to be the only kid there who's wearing his mother's shoes."

"Yeah, well, consider yourself lucky. Your mom rocks. Doc Martens? The other moms are duds."

Later that evening as I waited in line to pick him up, I watched the groups of kids pouring out of the old building. They were just at that age before full-blown teenager years. Cotillion had strict rules regarding attire, and it was gratifying to see the girls dressed demurely. Nick walked out, laughing, with some boys. The boys were either ramrod thin and gawky or they still held the pudginess of childhood. Nick retained his softness then; he hadn't shot up tall yet and become his father.

"How was it?"

"It was good."

He told me about the leader, Mr. Harris, an older gentleman who explained the importance of etiquette. They learned some dance steps and rotated from partner to partner. Toward the end of the evening, Mr. Harris announced that they'd be doing one more dance. This time the boys were to approach someone of their choosing and politely request a spin.

There was a girl, Nancy, who lived at the end of our block. She and Nick had the same birthday. They weren't friends, but they knew each other. There were three girls in the family, and they all had the misfortune of being extremely overweight. It couldn't have been easy for her at events like this, squeezed into her party dress, feeling uncomfortable. The world is not gentle to girls like Nancy.

"So when it was time to ask the girls to dance, all the boys rushed to the prettiest ones, and I was gonna do the same thing, and then I saw Nancy standing against the wall. Everyone was ignoring her. I slowed down for a second and thought about it. Then it kind of made me mad. It wasn't fair, you know? I did something kind of freaky, Mom. I walked right up to Nancy and said, really loud, 'Miss, would you do me the honor of joining me for a dance?' I said it loud because I wanted to show all the boys what jerks they were. Everyone kind of looked at me, but I didn't care."

"You did good, Boyo. You did just fine." I made a quick left turn so he wouldn't see me tear up.

Freaky, all right. Beautifully, breathtakingly freaky.

Nick saw his first Bob Dylan concert at age two. By the time he was a teenager, he and his father had attended many of them. At one concert, when Nick was thirteen, they waited together out by the trailers at intermission with the die-hard fans. Nick wanted to catch a glimpse of Bob. Finally, Craig went back in, but Nick insisted on waiting.

Ten minutes later he burst into the stadium.

"Dad! I talked to him!"

Dylan had emerged from the trailer to return to the stadium. Nick stood, with a few stragglers, by the fence. The others all yelled "Bob! Bob!" Nick raised his hands above his head and began bowing, silently, as if to royalty. Bob Dylan turned and walked right up to Nick. He signed his T-shirt and shook his hand. He thanked Nick for coming.

"His hands were soft, Dad, like Grandma Bea's."

I have that T-shirt tucked away in a ziplock bag, kept safe for my boy.

Craig was trying to take charge, be the father, but none of the old rules applied. Lucy and Rose just tried to stay out of the line of fire, free of being collateral damage. I kept trying to keep things calm. One morning—after Nick had run out, smashing through Craig's hand-made screen door and destroying it—we woke to find this letter pinned to the bedroom door:

Dear Pop,

I want to apologize for my behavior the other night. I did not realize my actions would affect you personally. I did not mean to hurt you, and after everything, and the time that had passed I realize how it could have been betraying your love, friendship and faith in me. I really regret that it created space and tension between us. I was enjoying the recent reconstruction of our friendship, and I really would like you to know that I need it right now. You don't understand what is going through my life right now. I am a stressed, depressed and confused mess that is inconsistent in my moods and behavior. I am dealing with tension, whether it is drug use, desire, or my attempt at motivating myself. I am also, I think, in love with Jenny, and it is a constant confusing roller coaster. Please maybe just wave a hand "hello" when I walk by around the house.

Love,
Nick

The "wave a hand 'hello'" makes me cry every single time.

At seventeen, he abandoned any pretense of going to school and moved into an apartment with his friend Jenny. They had been pals in high school. The plan was for him to work for me in my decorative painting business—he was still a skilled painter—and figure out what he wanted to do with his life. We'd all be happier at home without him, peace at last, and once he had full responsibility for his life, I was sure he'd wake up.

Yep, well, it went a little more like this: Without *any* supervision, his drug use expanded exponentially. He almost never showed up to work, prompting several incidents with me pounding on the door of his apartment, yelling, or honking my horn until one of his neighbors would threaten to call the police.

His lapses in performance at work would result in pay demotions. I was too afraid to actually fire him; I didn't know what he'd do. I knew I should go with tough love and let him take the consequences of his actions, because that's what everyone on talk radio said. Friends would ask me if I had tried this or that approach, but no one seemed to get it. Their helpful advice applied to a completely different world. I had long since lost the ability to exercise tough love. All I knew was fear. My entire world was a rickety house of cards—like the kind I used to build with my cousins as a kid—and instead of figuring out what was wrong, I just kept adding more cards. Like it wasn't going to fall.

I recently found a letter he had written after he hadn't showed up to the job.

Dear Mom,

I know this was my own fault and I reaped my own results in being a loser, stoned out like a moron. My self-destruction was a career of four slow years, which could explain my slow fucking recovery. It is such a frustration in my life, not remembering the good times, just a black spot that stained my existence.

I have improved and moved away from my near insanity and the suicidal tendencies that plagued my every day. I hope you see how hard it is to be me, inside my shoes, accepting what I've done to myself.

I hate my existing environment and yearn to be granted a chance at being who I am again and going away to art school.

Once I am reinstated into the environment that works for me, I will be a leader and contributing force in my field for that is my obligation to mankind to create beauty.

Until then, I beg that you bear with my bullshit, because I am rooting out the parasites and weeds until one day I won't ever go back. I want to take care of you and spoil you because I know you've sacrificed so much to support this family and myself.

Love and respect,
Nick

How could I have read words like *suicide* and *insanity* without alarms ringing? I don't even remember this letter. Where was I?

Nick and Jenny invited us over for dinner to see how they'd fixed up the place. Nick spent the entire time sitting silent on the couch, staring at an empty corner of the room. Jenny chatted uncomfortably with us as we slowly chewed our salad and chicken at the table. We left shortly after eating.

"Miriam, something is seriously wrong with him," Craig said as we walked to the car.

"I am going to call Cedars tomorrow. They have a solid psychiatric program. Maybe we can get some answers there."

A few days later, Jenny called me. "Mimi, Nick is acting really weird. I mean, really. Can you come over here?"

I walked in to find him sitting at the kitchen table, staring intently at the wood.

"He's been like this for about two hours. He won't talk, and he hasn't moved."

"Nick. Nickboy." I placed my palm on the middle of his back. "Why don't you come with Jenny and me. Let's go over to the hospital. Let's go to Kaiser and see if they can help you."

Without speaking, he got up and went to the car.

At Kaiser, a doctor took him into a private room, evaluated him, then decided an involuntary psychiatric hold was justified. The caveat was that I, as his legal guardian and a supposedly sane person, could decide to take him home.

I made a mistake of such gargantuan proportions that I will never forgive myself. I remember crouching against a wall outside of the hospital with Jenny. We had gone out to get some air, try to clear our heads. Cars whizzed by on Sunset; it was rush hour, incongruously scented by the buns baking at the Subway sandwich shop behind us. The boy who had been the most popular boy in high school was lying, almost catatonic, in a bed a few floors above us. I could feel him up there like I could feel my own bones. It was my job to figure out what to do. I asked Jenny a lot of questions about what drugs he had been using. It was shocking—everything from cold medicine to pot to LSD. I asked her about the specifics of his behavior. What *exactly* had been going on?

Any single thing she told me should have been enough to convince me to leave him at the hospital. She described all-night painting frenzies, relentless attempts to seduce her, bouts of paranoia. And yet, in the face of all that, I had only one overwhelming instinct: to not have him hospitalized. That, to me, felt like failure. My failure. It seems the same magic that enables a mother to find the superhuman strength to lift a car off her child can also propel her to become the superhero of fools.

Some nights, lying in bed, I draw an alternate scenario. One where I leave him at the hospital. He gets impeccable care. They're so smart, those doctors, they figure it all out. They realize he was developing schizophrenia and extend his hold to several weeks. As a result of the elimination of drugs and alcohol from his system, and the addition of an excellent nutritional regimen, he steers off his collision course with mental illness and on to a wonderful life. He grows up to be a famous artist. He marries a beautiful woman and has kids. His life is everything we all expected, and more.

Except that I checked him out of the hospital and he moved back home. I couldn't accept even the *possibility* of mental illness back then. I was still blaming drugs. I was operating in a stupor of denial. I wish someone had slapped me across the face and said, "Wake up!" So much time would pass before that slap arrived.

Craig and I had been dreaming for years about finding and buying some land at a good price, something entirely different from Larchmont Village, a place where we could eventually retire. One day, it occurred to me that might be a place where Craig could go away and work, and that would give me the time to help Nick as only I could. I started pushing the idea.

Craig went on several expeditions and eventually found five gorgeous acres in rural Washington state, with a big barn and a half-built house. It was driving distance from Scarlett, so we would be able to spend time with the grandchildren. Home prices in LA had skyrocketed, and we had a good amount of equity. We were able to obtain a line of credit from our house in Larchmont Village and bought the property. Craig would divide his time between Onalaska, Washington, and LA, leaving me the opportunity to control everything at home. I would no longer have to cope with two men.

He was excited about the new house project and loved being up there. In the summers, when I'd go up with the girls, we'd camp out at the house. We went to the lake, hiked, and explored, and after dinner we'd play board games. Without Nick, we could function like a regular family. We had something that felt normal and steady and, well, relaxed for a change. We had laughter. We had banter.

That's right. I would leave my son in LA—on his own, knowing the risks—for a few weeks of pretending. I am not emotionally limber enough to even try to justify it. I just have to live with the knowledge that I did in fact do that.

The part I didn't see at the time was how the girls perceived Craig's activities, especially Rose. She was still such a little girl that all she really knew was that her father had left her. That's how it felt. I was so busy with her brother I didn't see the darkness gathering around Rose.

I remember a movie I saw years ago where a woman backed confidently down her driveway, only to be obliterated by an oncoming truck. It was filmed in such a dramatic, breathtaking way that it stayed with me for a long time. I started having little episodes of anxiety, my breath just catching for a second, eyes darting to one side. I developed an odd twitch in my neck. I became jittery. I grew increasingly sure the truck was coming.

We continued to search for answers. After exhausting the drug rehabilitation programs, we were referred to a psychologist who thought Nick was suffering from depression and would benefit from medication. He referred us to Dr. Hamill, a young guy doing his psychiatric residency.

Dr. Hamill was tall and athletic, with a slightly crooked nose. He leaned his elbows on his desk and squinted at Nick. Craig and I were seated in two low armchairs off to the side. I should say here that mental illness is like a gale-force hurricane that blows through your life, leaving anything not bolted down gone. But it's not without its lighter moments.

"What do you have in mind for your treatment here, Nick?" asked Dr. Hamill.

"Oh, I was thinking of an office with couches and a big desk. A lot of wood. Oriental carpets would be nice, and messy bookshelves full of books."

Craig and I looked at each other. What the hell? Dr. Hamill nodded evenly, with a look of complete bewilderment. Nick leaned forward and put his elbows on the desk.

"Yeah, I'm also thinking corduroy. You know, one of those corduroy jackets with leather patches on the elbows. That's what the doctor should wear. Yeah. Jewish, for sure. Maybe a Woody

Allen–type guy. That's it. That's what I want! Don't forget the oriental carpets."

Craig and I looked at each other again. *Nick was art directing his therapy.*

Dr. Hamill took a special interest in Nick. Right off the bat, he prescribed an array of vitamin supplements that would be good for Nick's brain. We all worked together to figure this thing out. It finally felt like we were making some progress.

At the beginning of October, Nick turned eighteen, and the balance of power shifted; we could no longer force him to accept treatment. Our only leverage would be the roof over his head, and we didn't dare consider taking that away. What would become of him then? Each day he remained compliant was a gift.

Later in October, I received a birthday card from him. It was a family tradition to make all our own cards. This one was filled with creepy, slightly sexual drawings he'd done in ballpoint pen. Sunken-eyed old men with bony fingers. Half-naked women with their organs dripping out of their stomachs. Carefully shaded drops of blood emerging from mouths, eyes. Inside he wrote:

> As your growing son of 18, I take pleasure in glorifying your bitter gingersnap of a smile. One could read your 48 years of mannerisms endlessly enthralled and hypnotized into a frozen Dali moment of infinity.

I tried so hard to dismiss the card as *creative* or just the work of a teenager trying to push the boundaries. But I couldn't. I called Dr. Hamill. After seeing it, he confirmed that the card was indeed alarming. It indicated another level of seriousness. He suggested Nick begin seeing him twice a week.

"I can't believe he would give me a card like that," I said to Dr. Hamill over the phone.

"As we go forward, Mimi, there will be times when you have to remember it is the disease talking, not Nick." Hearing this made me realize nothing was ever going to be the same again.

October in Los Angeles usually comes with one last exhale of summer. It can get very warm, the Santa Ana winds blowing their fiery breath through the city. I was working on a large-scale mural for a restaurant in our neighborhood, painting after hours and through the night so they didn't have to close down entirely. Craig was up in Washington and the girls were at home.

I liked this kind of project, just me alone with the paint. The evening had turned balmy, and I was happy for a minute.

It was about ten o'clock when my phone rang—Dr. Hamill. I climbed down from the scaffold and went out back to the alley to talk. Man, it was beautiful out. Sparkling lights against an almost-night sky, warm wind on my skin. Dr. Hamill told me he had a diagnosis for Nick: bipolar disorder. By then I knew all the different conditions, and no description was necessary.

"He is going to have to go on medication," he said.

"What kind of medication?"

"The medication for bipolar is quite effective. Nick can live a normal life if he stays with it. I'd like to start with Abilify."

"What else can we do?"

"You have to prepare yourself for the possibility that it could also be schizophrenia," the good doctor told me. "But let's not get ahead of ourselves, now. Let's treat it as bipolar. There is every reason to be optimistic."

The doctor's words were like physical things; each consonant brought the sting of a small insect, vowels the wallop of a punch. It was not a final diagnosis. It could change. There was a spectrum of mental illnesses, and a patient's place on it is fluid.

I could feel the blood rushing in my body along with a thousand ferocious thoughts. It was official. My son was mentally ill.

I did what I always do. I went inside and finished my work. I did a good job. When the walls had their second coat, I went to the laundry sink and carefully washed my brushes. I tapped the ferrule of each one on the tip of my boot to knock out excess water. I removed the roller covers from the handles and washed them all. I walked the site to make sure I hadn't forgotten anything, spilled any paint. I turned out the lights. I locked the door. I set the alarm.

3

THE MEDICATION WARS

Nick did not want to go on medication. "Dr. Hamill is wrong," he said. "I am not sick." This is a common reaction. Now that he was eighteen, we couldn't force him to continue treatment. Calmly, reasonably, we explained that the drugs would simply correct a chemical imbalance in his brain and he would feel better. The anxiety and depression would be lessened, and his life would improve. Dr. Hamill tried to diminish the stigma, showing him literature and videos, normalizing the issue. I sat with a demented grin on my face and blathered about famous creative people who had mental illnesses.

"Isaac Newton, Nick! Brian Wilson from the Beach Boys! The artist Edvard Munch! Vincent van Gogh! Ted Turner, who is very famous and successful, *he* is bipolar! Patty Duke . . . it didn't ruin *her* career! For God's sake, Winston Churchill, who is your father's sixth cousin, *he* had depression *and* possible bipolar! And *he* saved all the Jews from Hitler! That's right, *your* relatives!"

In the end, we paid Nick to take the medication. I know this goes against everything we all have been taught about parenting, but I have a note from my doctor. That's right, Dr. Hamill told us to forget the conventional wisdom. What mattered, all that mattered, was to get Nick on the medicine. The sooner he was on it, the less damage to his still-developing brain, the more hope for a good outcome. *A good outcome.* This was a phrase I had never used before, and then it became a mantra.

Every day in the kitchen, I would give him his meds and ten dollars. His sisters were appalled. No one had ever, even once, offered them money to take their amoxicillin. Mom had disappointed them beyond belief, and she didn't have anything near a plausible explanation. They knew about Nick's diagnosis, but really, to all of us, it still seemed unreal. We still thought this incursion was temporary. After all, once the fourteen-day course of amoxicillin ended, everything was fine.

I was still a novice at being the medicine police. Incredible, now, to admit this, but it never occurred to me that Nick wasn't swallowing the tablets—"cheeking it," as I now know it's called. I had seen *One Flew Over the Cuckoo's Nest* and thought it was a great movie. I, like everyone else, saw Nurse Ratched as the villain. The rebellious McMurphy was my hero; Martini and Chief Bromden were his oddball cohorts. They were just misunderstood and unappreciated by the rigid "normal" world.

The book *Surviving Schizophrenia* by E. Fuller Torrey, MD (HarperCollins, 2000) is regarded as the standard reference book on the disease. For me, it's the bible. In the back of the book, he has a section called "50 of the Best and 15 of the Worst Books on Schizophrenia." Imagine my dismay to see the book on which the movie is based, *One Flew Over the Cuckoo's Nest* by Ken Kesey, listed by Dr. Torrey as one of the worst. His point is this: the patients are depicted as oppressed, not sick, as McMurphy tries to mobilize them to challenge the evils of the state hospital. In the end, Chief Bromden escapes to live happily ever after outside the facility. In reality, he probably would have joined the legions of the homeless who live under bridges and in alleys.

It is a fact that marijuana can disrupt the chemistry of developing brains. I am convinced that Nick's drug use exacerbated his schizophrenia. There are theories that schizophrenia might not have even developed had he not routinely abused these drugs. When I reach realizations like this, I have to face the truth about my hiding. I wasn't just cloaking our secrets from the outside world, I was hiding them from myself. Even with my bruised memory, I can see the damage done.

Nick's behavior didn't improve. Of course, that was because he wasn't taking the medication, but I didn't know that yet. Agitated and combative, he started stealing, taking what he wanted from the girls' rooms, my purse.

Lucy ran into the kitchen crying, sat at the table, and said, "I have to tell you something terrible."

"What is it?"

"Mom . . ." She couldn't talk. She just held her head in her hands.

"Lucy, please, you're scaring me."

"I went into your room to use your bathroom, and Nick was in there. He was over by the window seat." At this she started wailing. "He was stealing money from your purse!"

This was so unthinkable, so impossible, that it shook her to the core. In a million years she couldn't imagine stealing money from her mother.

"What is happening, Mom? How could he do this?"

I had no answer for her that wouldn't make it all worse.

I bought each of the girls a decorative trunk to keep their *special* things in, each with its own padlock. We had a firm family policy about no locks on doors, so this was the only way to protect their things.

My doctor had given me a prescription for Xanax, just for the short term, to help with my stress management. One day I opened my bathroom drawer, and it was not there. I had hidden it way in the back, but it was gone. Could I have moved it? After tearing my bathroom and bedroom completely apart, I knew Nick must have gotten to it.

"Nick!" I called. "Come up here."

I faced him in a chair.

"All right, Bub. I know what you did." He peered at me innocently. "I am going to give you one chance to come clean. If you tell me the truth, there will be no consequences, but if you lie to me now, all hell is going to break loose."

Our eyes locked, and I waited.

He sang like a canary.

Sitting there, I listened to a breathless litany of transgressions committed over the years that would curl a priest's toenails. Stuff I had no idea about. And it kept coming. It ranged from the small-time to the reckless and even petty criminal. It still keeps me awake at night. He confessed every bad thing he had ever done but denied taking the pills. I don't know which was worse, the fact that I had granted him impunity ahead of time or that it turned out he didn't steal the damn pills after all.

Years later, looking for an earring, I found the expired Xanax in my jewelry box.

Sometimes Nick would blow up at the girls, and that was the worst. Once we arrived home with hamburgers, and not knowing he was there, we hadn't gotten him one. He asked Lucy for a bite. She gave him the burger, and he took a huge chunk out of it. She complained, and he picked up all the food and threw it against the wall.

Now, one would expect a lot of yelling and fighting to follow, but not in our house. We had already adjusted to the new normal and immediately prioritized the issues. Yes, Nick was wrong to have splattered the food across the kitchen. Yes, Lucy was justified in being upset. But what was the biggest issue we *all* knew we had to contend with first? Dad.

A little background: Craig had built an exquisite kitchen that was his crowning glory as a woodworker, and he was, understandably, protective of it. But he had unreasonable expectations that nothing would ever sully it. An entire dinner of In-N-Out was way over the line. Crazy or not, even Nick knew that the first damage-control issue was upstairs watching the evening news.

"What's going on down there?" Craig yelled from the bedroom.

Nick, Lucy, Rose, and I looked at each other with wide eyes and set in motion a stealth cleanup mission that was completed within seconds of Craig coming down the stairs. We looked up innocently and said, "Huh? What?"

It was almost funny. In fact, when the girls and I tell the story to each other these days, we do laugh. It seems funny. But it wasn't. It was like we were at war, living in such a heightened state of readiness, always wary of the next possible blowup. Lucy should have been able to get mad at her brother and express her indignation. Rose just wanted to eat her burger. Nick was hearing voices, but the girls had lost theirs. No one was listening to anyone.

Rose just kept shrinking and shrinking, staying out of the way. Nick's behavior became more and more disturbing. Craig and I continually clashed, and those two girls endured. They still seemed fine. They did well in school and had friends. There was laughter and happiness in our lives, but what must it have been like to grow up in a world where the ground beneath you was constantly shifting? I don't really have to ask that question. I know. They have told me.

Behind my front door lived something unfathomable and singular. I stared out my windows at the neighborhood like it was one of those puzzles where you circle words as you see them in the block of letters. While some families were dealing with drug problems or bad behavior, no one ever discussed mental illness. Perfect Larchmont Village continued its rubric of daily life without the O'Rourke family. All I wanted was to know I wasn't the only one. Something to indicate that I wasn't absolutely alone.

The thing that people don't understand is that the crazy isn't constant. We could go weeks without an incident. During those times, I was sure the medication was working. I had been told that a person with bipolar could live a normal life. I dismissed evidence I shouldn't have in order to maintain hope. I can see that now.

Around this time something kind of wonderful happened. A client whose house I had painted in Los Angeles asked us to paint murals in her new apartment in Paris. Craig and I would go, and we decided to bring Nick along. We saw this as an opportunity to get him out of his surroundings, get some of that old "perspective" I kept thinking was the cure for mental illness. The three of us could paint together, perhaps rediscover our connection to each other, to art.

Nick had been living in a guesthouse around the corner. I had negotiated a six-month lease in order to get him out of the house. The six months were up; perfect timing. After spending the weekend packing up, he dropped his things off at our house and said, "It's all good."

"What does that mean, 'It's all good'?" I asked.

"It means I cleaned the whole place up and everything is fine."

"Really? I don't even have to go over there and check?"

"Nope."

Even without the crazy, I knew better than that. I had a housekeeper, Maria, who came once a week. It was her day, so we loaded up the car with supplies. I knew it wouldn't be clean, but I wasn't ready for what we found. I'll never forget poor Maria's face. It was that expression you see in horror movies when the actress realizes something *really* bad is going to happen to her. I was so ashamed. Old food and dishes covered the kitchen, the sink was clogged, the bathroom blanketed in green mold. My son lived like an animal, and now I had a witness. We were in it together now. After many hours of cleaning, Maria and I left, shell-shocked. We never spoke of it again. I still thought that if I didn't talk about it, it wouldn't be real. I didn't even confront Nick. There was no point.

When Craig asked me how bad it was, I said, "Not too bad."

I hired the grown daughter of my friend Brenda to stay with Lucy and Rose. They loved her and were excited to "be on their own." Nick seemed to be taking his medication and was excited to go. Craig bought a couple of berets, and off we went.

The time in Paris exists in parentheses. We painted, saw the sights. We ate lots of food. One night, in a small brasserie, Nick excused himself and went upstairs to the bathroom. He was gone a long time. "Maybe you'd better go up and check on him?"

In a couple of minutes, Craig came downstairs with an amused expression. "Oh, he's fine. Nothing to worry about there."

Nick came over, grabbed his jacket, and headed toward a stunning older girl waiting by the door. He disappeared with her for the night. He went to Jim Morrison's grave and spent the night smoking cigarettes and drinking wine. The next day, the three of us walked the Louvre and marveled at the paintings. We were immersed in all the things we all loved. It was fantastic.

"Look at our boy, charming the Parisian girls," I said.

"He's doing a good job at work, don't you think?" Craig replied.

"Totally," I said. "He's really trying hard."

"Spending the night at Jim Morrison's grave is something I would have done at that age." Craig grinned.

I smiled back. "He's so talented. He is a true artist. Maybe we're buying into all this mental illness stuff, and he's just an eccentric artist. We should've known better." I thought of the day before, the brush in Nick's hand moving across the wall of the apartment as we stenciled arabesques, a smile on his face.

"Yeah."

"Yeah."

Standing in front of a Byzantine sculpture, Craig looked like a slightly worn version of Nick with the same broad back. I found comfort in the ivory slope of a stone shoulder.

"Let's go look at some contemporary art!" Nick said.

"I'm not looking at any Jeff Koons," Craig replied.

"If I saw Jeff Koons in person, I would smack him," I said.

"Me too," Craig replied, deadpan.

"You guys are crazy," Nick said, smiling.

When the job was completed, Nick and I flew home together;

Craig had gone a day earlier. I was awakened by two flight attendants. They held his passport open and asked, "Do you know this person?" I have to admit that my initial impulse was to say no and go back to sleep.

"Yes." I stammered a little. "Why?"

"He has refused to stay in his assigned seat and repeatedly tried to sneak into the first-class section. The flight attendants are uneasy, and the passengers are being disturbed. If you will make sure he stays in his seat, we will return his passport."

"I'll take care of it. I'm sure it's just a misunderstanding," I said. "Misunderstanding" was becoming a distressingly common word in my vocabulary.

I walked quietly over to where Nick was seated.

"What the hell, Nick? You want to get kicked off the plane? You know it's a post-9/11 world, man. They don't take lightly to these kinds of hijinks."

"Oh, they overreacted," he said. That was his default reply when reprimanded, when I would find his carpet burned in a thousand places by cigarettes or three weeks of garbage in the refrigerator. Everybody was always overreacting.

"Really? Well, put your passport in your pocket and your ass in that seat. It's the middle of the night. Behave yourself, buddy." I turned and headed back to my place.

In a loud whisper he said, "There's a bunch of seats up there. I don't know why they care anyway."

I gave him my best mom stink eye. Sometime later I awoke to see not only the two flight attendants but the actual copilot staring down at me.

The copilot said sternly, "We have a serious problem here, ma'am. Your son will not stay in his seat. We have confiscated his passport and will turn him over to the authorities when we reach Los Angeles."

I looked the pilot in the eye and said, "You know what? He's eighteen. Do what you want. I'm going to sleep." The effort of keeping the facade up, convincing myself Nick's problems were temporary, pushing down my own fear . . . had worn me down. At that moment I had nothing left.

Not my finest hour.

I'm not sure what transpired during the rest of the flight, but when I woke up Nick was in his seat, holding his passport, a smile on his face. I asked him what had happened.

"Oh, the flight attendant and I have an understanding."

"What does that mean? You got your passport back?" I was relieved but also feeling a little like a monster for abandoning him.

"Yeah," Nick said. "I just talked to him and explained things, and we're fine."

This is an interesting component of the disease. As Nick got crazier and crazier, he still was able to call on his ability to charm people when necessary. He could spend an entire day with me and not utter a word, only nod. Later on the very same day, when we find ourselves at the Subway counter, all of a sudden he is articulate, describing the sandwich he wants.

"I'd like the carved turkey on a whole wheat roll. No thank you, I don't want it toasted."

"Really?" I ask the heavens.

"And please put the mayonnaise on both sides. Can I get extra onions and olives? Thank you so much."

You can ask him a thousand questions and get only a thousand grunts, but if he believes I've shorted him on his daily money, I find myself dealing with an accountant.

"No, Mom. You gave me an extra five on Tuesday. It's been two days. We are back to ten now," he'd litigate.

"Nick, I also gave you an extra pack of cigarettes. You're forgetting that," I'd counter.

"That was *last* week. I made that up by taking only five over the weekend."

Eventually, I'd give in. Or give up. The thing is, I didn't remember all those details. He could have been telling the truth.

The more important issue was not my inability to hold firm but his ability to persevere in his agenda. It made me wonder what else was still in there, dormant, waiting for the requisite moment to emerge. Couldn't we just find some damn way to scrape off this pesky mental illness and free him?

After Paris, Nick moved back into the house; he had nowhere else to go. He got money from odd jobs and painting work he did with friends. We had moved to a larger house on Norton, two blocks from our old one, when Nick was nine. He'd gotten the best bedroom, the one with a balcony. Now we gave him the TV room because none of us wanted him upstairs. Craig began to stay at "the farm," as we were optimistically calling it, a lot of the time. Me? I still thought I was going to be able to clear up the Nick Problem if everyone would just get out of my way. At this point that belief was based upon nothing more than momentum.

I continued my policy of nondisclosure and cover-up. That helped. It meant that Craig didn't ask questions anymore. A transformation was occurring in and around Nick's room; his crazy was filling the place up. He was collecting a strange mélange of discarded furniture from garage sales and curbsides. He put a lock from Craig's shop on the door. I removed the lock. He put another one on. This continued for the entire year. The girls were beside themselves. *No locks were allowed.* Once again, I had betrayed them with my inconsistent parenting.

My so-called parenting. It definitely had devolved from the time we lived on Ridgewood, when I envisioned myself as the perfect Larchmont mom. But even back then, I had my moments. I remembered one incident in particular, when Nick was eight.

Lucy and Nick would not stop fighting. She kept knocking over the towers he was making. She was having a ball. He was not amused.

Rose was an infant then, and my main priority was keeping her asleep.

"Will you two stop it? If you wake up the baby, I will be very upset."

Carefully, Nick began a new tower of the green rectangular blocks with the cutout arch. Within minutes, I heard a loud crash and screaming. Stomping back into the room, I demanded quiet, but by then it was a dogfight.

I guess because Nick was bigger and hitting Lucy, I impulsively pulled him into the kitchen.

"What did I ask? One thing. To be quiet."

"She kept knocking over my buildings. This isn't fair."

"You are the older one, and I expect you to set an example!" I snapped. "This is unacceptable!" Now I was yelling. I took his arm and spanked him on the butt until I realized what I was doing and stopped, horrified. Craig and I didn't spank our kids.

I sent him to his room. The bay window distorted my reflection, and I saw a beast.

With a long inhale, I walked to Nick's room. Sitting cross-legged on his bed, he looked plaintively at me.

"Nick, I want to apologize. I lost my temper. It was wrong for you to hit Lucy, but I shouldn't have spanked you. That was even more wrong."

His inky brown eyes met mine. "It's okay, Mom. I understand. I'm just worried about *you*. I've never seen you like that."

It felt like the sprinkling down of pebbles in some brook in the forest. It felt like the first few drops of a great rain. I saw it then—*he understood more than I did*.

"Why don't you go lie down in Rose's room until she wakes up?" he said. "I'll be nice to Lucy now, Mom. I'll keep her quiet."

I sat on the edge of my bed looking at the closed door, stunned by his uncomplicated wisdom. I felt safe under the supervision of my eight-year-old son.

Nick still held his friends in thrall during the time he was losing his mind. They looked to him for guidance and ideas, most of which he had learned at Craig's knee. Ferlinghetti, Pablo Neruda, Coltrane—no one else's parents had introduced these artists to them. To his friends, Nick was brilliant; as he started to get crazy, more brilliant.

After we returned from Paris, he decided to make an art studio for himself in the driveway. He worked on large-scale, elaborate projects with his friends until late in the night, playing loud music and not doing any of his chores. He came and went as he pleased, now openly refusing to take his meds. The girls began to regard me with a new mixture of disgust and resentment.

They started to take care of each other.

Lucy, Rose, and I sat at the dinner table. It looked like the classic American dinner hour, minus father and brother. Everyone had washed their hands. Before us was a lovely meal, made from scratch. Roast chicken, vegetables, salad. Plates to pass with a smile and pass again. Buster slept with his girth smashed against the glass door. Suddenly, the whole backyard was illuminated, lit in a blinding burst, aglow with countless string lights. Four teenage boys of varying sizes were in the process of covering their naked bodies in paint. As the three of us sat agape, they proceeded to roll around on big swaths of fabric.

Then the music began, crashing and screaming guitar riffs, electronic vibrations, shattering noises I couldn't even identify. Through the sliding glass door, we stared at our overlit backyard filled with noise, chaos, and adolescent penises flapping in the breeze. I didn't have enough hands to cover all the eyes and ears.

The girls were laughing, covering their own eyes, as I ran out back to put a stop to the display.

The next morning, I insisted to Nick that he get a job. This would force him into some semblance of a schedule, require accountability, and ultimately bring back the boy I had known.

"Okay, Ma, that's a good idea. I could use some money. Maybe I can get my job back at American Rag. I liked that job."

"That might work. Do you still know anyone there?"

"I'm not sure, but I'll go over and see."

Nick did go to the store and attempt to apply for a job. There were no openings. He proceeded to barrage the woman in charge of hiring with phone calls, letters, and drop-ins, refusing to take no for an answer. I'd raised my kids with a strong work ethic and a philosophy of not giving up, so I could see what he was trying to do. In Nick's intense interpretation of that philosophy, what the good people at American Rag saw was a stalker.

I received a call from my friend Jean, who was dating the owner of the store.

"I really don't know how to get into this, but do you know that Nick has been trying to get a job over at American Rag?" she asked.

"Yes, I did know that. But he told me there were no openings."

"It's a little more complicated than that," she said.

There was the tightness in my chest again, the feeling that we were about to be obliterated by that damn truck.

"It seems he is harassing the manager to the degree that she's starting to feel unsafe. I'm so sorry to have to tell you this, Mimi. I feel terrible."

"No, no. Don't apologize," I said. "I appreciate you giving me the heads-up. Sometimes he's a little overzealous, you know. I'm sure it's just a *misunderstanding*."

I decided that breathing for a minute might be a good idea. What had she actually said, anyway? He was being persistent in his attempt to find a job. This was a good thing. I'd just talk to him, tell him I was proud he was trying but maybe it was time to look elsewhere.

Later that day, when he at last wandered in, I caught him before he could retreat into his room. "Nick, I know you are being tenacious in your attempt to get your job back at American Rag, and I think that's great."

"Yeah, I think the lady likes me. I'm just trying to convince her."

"Well, there comes a point where you have to back off and let the person make their decision. If you appear too eager, it can backfire."

"Okay, sure."

Silently retreating into his nascent madness, he closed the door. Nothing more was mentioned for a week.

It was early. I had just gotten the girls off to school when my phone rang. It was Jean again.

"Mimi, I'm so sorry, but I just heard that Nick is outside the store demanding to see the manager, and they are going to call the police if you don't get him out of there." She sounded so distressed, I felt the urge to comfort *her*.

Hanging up the phone, I realized that this time there was no time for breathing. What do I do? Craig, of course, was in Washington. I called Nick's phone and left an incoherent message. I knew I should get in the car and go look for him, but I didn't want to do it alone. I called my close friend Jill, who lived around the corner.

"Jill. It's me. I need help."

In my adult life, I don't think I had ever just outright asked for help. Ever. In one quick minute, she was at my house. We drove over to the store in her car. He was nowhere to be found. I was sure he had been arrested. We called Jean, and she said he had gone away on his own. A small blessing. Jill drove me all around, searching, a couple of housewife spies in pajamas. We spotted him once but then lost him. Finally, we went home, me calling him over and over all the way.

"Should I come in and wait with you?"

I already had the passenger side open and one foot out the door.

"Oh, no. I'm fine. You need to go to work. Thank you so much for helping me. I just couldn't face it alone." I went into the house.

Nick was inside, eating breakfast, as nonchalant as can be. I pulled up my chair to the table. I cleared my throat and asked him to look up for a moment, please. I needed to speak with him. I warned him about the trouble he would get into if he ever showed his face at American Rag again. I addressed the troubling content of the letters he'd written to the manager, which Jean had given to me. They weren't threatening at all; instead, they were earnest in a very old-fashioned way. But there was something—something between the lines—that was disquieting.

By this time, when under stress or even at relaxed moments, he had begun to use language in ways that could no longer be attributed to some sense of art or poetic license or original self-expression. His communication was now frequently bizarre and incomprehensible. What had once been subtle and intermittent and even charming was now a regular feature of his disease.

"Ma, certain ulmighty truth and fiction can reiterate a strengthy relationship," he said as he finished eating. Outside the window, hovering just over his head, I noticed how a jagged branch suddenly looked like lightning in the sky.

I called Jean to tell her he wouldn't bother them again. She was one of those women who was always perfectly put together: hair, nail polish, makeup. It felt like we were of two different species. Through the whole incident, she treated me with kindness and understanding. I mean, this was an awful situation. We lived in a neighborhood where people cared a lot about appearances. She never once made me feel anything near embarrassment. Nick stopped going to the store, and Jean never mentioned it again.

There was a game we played when we were kids, at slumber parties. One of us would lie on the floor on her back. Everyone would gather around, kneeling, and put two fingers from either hand underneath her. At the agreed-upon moment, all the girls would lift the prone one lightly up into the air, as though she were a feather. Just two fingers from each hand of every girl, and there was magic. That's what women do.

The TV room/driveway/backyard art extravaganza was uncontainable. Nick's coterie of eccentrics was there all hours of the day and night.

He set up work tables on the lawn, kids slept on the back porch, and food disappeared at a fantastical rate. He wouldn't allow any of us into his room. He'd clean up his act when Craig came home. There was some part of him that craved Craig's approval so strongly it seemed to overpower his illness. I continued to hide the insanity that ensued after his departure. With just a little more time I'd have this thing nailed down.

The girls liked the art scene. They were getting older, and having a bunch of cute outsider boys around was interesting. They'd hang around and flirt shamelessly, and so the boys in turn hung around indefinitely. It was a bacchanal of adolescent intrigue.

I was quite simply unable to exert any authority. My coping was then more of a "if you can't beat 'em, join 'em" mode. What I could alter was my own perception, and so I decided to believe that we had some quirky, cool thing going on. Screw all the uptight Larchmont neighbors! We here are artists. We have our own set of rules. I'd have a big glass of wine and reimagine my life into a flourish. I was at the center of a living mural, reclining on brightly colored embroidered pillows, harem style. All around me were young painters, musicians, engaged in the pursuit of art making. It was a fabulous delusion.

One day I was checking to make sure he'd locked the TV room window. A corner of a ziplock bag was poking out from under his mattress. I went over to it and pulled it out. The truth was now, actually, in my own two hands. I held a bag of psychedelic mushrooms. I understood then. Of course. They weren't a coterie of eccentrics; they were just a bunch of garden-variety druggies.

Naturally, given my desire to play spin doctor and continue to retail this cover story of—what?—teenage coming-of-age, I didn't tell Craig. I confronted Nick about the drugs, and, God help me, I let him convince me they weren't his. He fed me the drug that he knew I wanted: deniability. I flushed them down the toilet.

But it was the evidence of drug use under my roof that made me put my foot down on the household shenanigans. I couldn't allow drugs around Lucy and Rose, now that I was fully aware of their presence. I shut down the chaotic bohemian circus, which left Nick aimless and bored. His hapless associates went back to college or "whatever." The girls returned to school in the fall. They still got good grades, and I clung to that as the indicator of well-being.

I didn't know what to do with Nick. I had no control over him in terms of treatment or medication. I was hostage to a ruthless terror of what would happen to him if I were to really and truly kick him out of the house, so I decided to try to send him to college again. Now I certainly see that I'd begun to go mad myself. How did I think he'd gain admission, much less fare, in college?

I did some research. I sought out liberal nontraditional schools that might be able to give him some structure as well as some success and focus. I came upon Evergreen State College in Olympia, Washington. Evergreen has an interdisciplinary arts-oriented program geared to undergraduates who do not meet standard entrance requirements per se but show promise and talent by legitimate alternative measures. I called and had them send the application forms.

"Evergreen is in the book *Colleges that Change Lives*," I told him. "It's a really great college. On top of that, it has a fabulous art department. You'll even get to be near Dad. You can go visit on weekends!"

Filial devotion and longing were the incentives that cinched his decision to accept the offer. I filled out all the paperwork myself, and together we assembled an impressive portfolio. Nick wrote a letter pleading his case. *I know I have wasted so many chances, I want to make important art, please take a chance on me . . .* I gave it a glancing editorial eye. Once I removed the invented words, it actually read quite well. He made a persuasive case for himself. We slapped a stamp on it and hoped for the best.

A few weeks later, an envelope from Evergreen arrived. Nick stood in the foyer and nervously tore it open, then read it aloud.

"Dear Nick, we see great potential in you and have decided to offer you a place in our special admission program."

I was careful not to jinx everything by showing my boundless joy. The letter went on to explain the terms of his acceptance. He would be on probation for the first trimester and had to be monitored by a counselor.

"Well," I said tentatively, "what do you think? Need some time to think it over?"

"Are you kidding?" He slammed the paper down. "A real college wants me? I'm going!"

We called Craig and told him. We danced around. I tried to hug him, but he backed off. The girls' laughter was effervescent. Their brother was going to college.

Meanwhile, guilt washed over me. I knew it wasn't going to work. But at that point of absolute and desperate exhaustion, magical thinking took over. I needed relief and hope. As we prepared for his transition to school, Nick was obstinate and difficult about the actual process of packing up. He fought with me about every detail. He dug in his heels in some regressive rebellion. I had become the enemy.

"This is my life now, Ma, and you can't tell me what to do." I backed off, and somehow he assembled some belongings for his new life.

Two weeks before he was set to leave, he announced that his truck was packed, and he was going to spend some time on the road, maybe stop and visit Scarlett on the way up.

"Then I am going to stay with my dad. He gets me."

4

THE SLAP

I remember so much of this epic in excruciating detail, it clutches my poor brain in the moments before sleep. Oddly, there are also large parts that remain a blur, like a shaken-up snow globe slowly settling. The weeks between Nick's departure and return are of the snow-globe variety, only there is no snow, no glitter—just pieces of our lives crashing slowly through liquid.

The girls and I stood in the driveway and waved goodbye, just like regular people. When he was no longer in sight, we went inside and together immediately began dismantling the Cray Room, as we called the TV room at that point. What we found was shocking—old, crusty plates of food, things stolen from the girls' rooms, used condoms. I ended up throwing away every single thing. I even tore out the carpet.

I painted the ceiling a pale French blue and the walls a calm beige. I replaced the carpet with beige. I got a beige couch. It must be explained here that beige has a very specific meaning in our family. Craig and I are color people. Lots of color. And if a wall is to be light, then it is white, never beige. Beige represents everything we reject: conventionality, conformity, neutrality. Lucy and Rose watched the process play out, stupefied, as I transformed Nick's "Cray" cave into the equivalent of a doctor's waiting room. All I wanted to do was dislodge every piece of crazy from that room and Simonize it.

Somewhere between California and Washington, Nick got himself arrested. I believe marijuana and a belligerent attitude toward the officers were the causes. He spent the night in jail and somehow was released, albeit without his driver's license, the next morning.

The plan to spend some meaningful length of time with his father lasted a mere two days. Nick had arrived in Washington very angry at me. He spent most of the first day deriding me to Craig.

"Mimi, he was calling you disgusting names, saying you lie about him and make up stories to turn me against him!"

After that, he evidently stayed in his room, drinking and smoking. Nick has a fantastic ability to burrow into a space and very quickly make it into his own world, daunting to others.

"What am I supposed to do? He won't come out. How the hell is he going to go to *college*?" Craig was out in the barn, beside himself.

"It's going to work. We just have to get him through another week."

"You know, I think you are the one who's insane, Feldman."

"I really think that if we can just get him started, he could rise to the occasion. If he stays on his meds, it's possible."

"You're dreaming."

"Please, Craig. Please try. I don't know what else to do." I was begging him, actually, truthfully as much for my own sake, and his, as it was for Nick.

The next day Craig gave him an ultimatum about his conduct at the house. Nick loaded up his truck and drove off in a grinding snarl of gravel and rain.

It was a beautiful day in Malibu. I was visiting friends and enjoying life for a precious minute. Then my phone rang.

"Mom, I don't know what to do. Dad kicked me out for no reason at all, and I have nowhere to go," Nick reported.

"Wait, what?" Those two words had become my own personal jingle.

"I'm in Tumwater. They won't rent me a motel room because the police kept my license, and I don't know what to do."

"Tumwater, what are you . . . wait, what? The police?"

"It wasn't my fault, Ma. I was just burning some Nag Champa in my car"—because *everyone* burns incense in their car—"and these stupid hick police thought it was pot. Can you believe it?"

Well, yes, I could believe it. About that time my chest was contracting in a way that corresponded dangerously with public service commercials about heart attacks. I listened to a saga involving, of course, a lot of misunderstandings and overreacting.

My friends were in the beach house enjoying the afternoon, surely wondering where I was. I was crouched on the parkway outside, hissing like a deranged person into my flip phone. I found a motel in Tumwater and convinced them to rent him a room on my credit card.

"Just go to the motel, check in, and don't get into any trouble," I instructed.

Tanned surfers sped by in beat-up station wagons. A Lamborghini, parked nearby, shined in the sun. The sky was cloudless. I could see the beach and the turquoise water; I just couldn't get there. I jammed the cell phone between my cheek and shoulder as I rummaged in my purse for a pen. I began to foresee the possibility of real disaster ahead.

All I wanted in this life was to jump into the beckoning ocean. Throw my body up against the powerful waves or dive smoothly through them. What I didn't want to do was talk to Craig about our insane son. I decided to postpone the conversation and call him on the way home. Walking back to my friends on the shore, I smiled and shoved the credit card in my pocket.

All the pieces in the snow globe were far from settling yet. The next week was a blur of phone calls, arguments, and arrangements. Nick was in the motel waiting it out until he could move into the dorm. Craig was furious, despondent, and feeling guilty.

Somehow, Nick's driver's license was mailed to Craig, who drove all the way up to his motel to give it to him. Nick refused to open the door. God only knows what was going on in there. After about forty-five minutes, Craig slid it under the door and left.

"Oh, well, that's good, so now he has his license. He'll need that when school starts." I was a case study of denial.

The next we heard was that Nick had moved into his dorm. He was vague about the situation when we talked.

"I don't really like my roommates," he said. "They're a lot younger than me, and all they do is party."

"Just stay with the program. You'll find friends who suit you. How is the preregistration going?"

"I like my counselor, and there are a lot of art classes."

After conversations like that, I'd chisel out a little niche of optimism. It was the Friday before the Monday when classes began. I held my breath.

I had gotten home from a jobsite. We were painting a large mural and the building was still under construction, as was often the case. I had my hard hat and steel-toed boots on, and was putting equipment away in the sheds. Craig was out working in the shop. I could hear the shrill whiz of the table saw, and the comforting aroma of sawdust hung in the air. I stayed in it, in a kind of bliss, holding on to the sensations. I put my gallons of paint away neatly on the shelves. As I was hanging the rollers up, I heard the droning voice of Bob Dylan singing "Forever Young" in my pocket. Lucy had put a specific ringtone on my phone for each kid.

"Mom, hi, it's Nick. Hi," he said quickly.

"Hey, Nick. Wow, school starts on Monday. Are you excited?" I asked.

"Yeah, I guess. I need to ask you something, Ma."

"Okay, what?"

"Who's my real father?"

"What are you talking about?"

"Mom, I know Dad's not my real father. It's Bob Dylan. I know it. You've been hiding it from me all this time, and I just want the truth."

The capacity we humans have to just shut down when things are too much is like the psychological equivalent of your body going into shock after losing a limb. "That's ridiculous. I've got a bunch of ladders to unload." I hung up and went back to work. I told no one. In those days, speaking things out loud made them real.

Later that night Nick called again. I let it go to voice mail.

On Saturday afternoon, Craig and I were at our favorite Mexican restaurant when he called again. This time I answered.

"Mom, you can't believe who I am looking at right now, right here in downtown Olympia!"

"Who?"

"It's Paul Simon! He's driving around in a Rolls-Royce. He must be here for a concert."

Well, at least he wasn't claiming Paul was his father. I mean, this was plausible. Paul Simon could be in Olympia. This didn't necessarily mean Nick was insane.

"That's cool. You all ready for school on Monday?"

"How does he sound?" Craig mouthed over tortilla chips. Ranchero music droned from the bar, and an old ceiling fan clacked above us.

"Kind of manic," I said, covering the phone.

"Yep. It's all good. Talk to you soon." Nick sounded racy, talking fast. I didn't mention the Bob Dylan thing.

Sunday began as most Sundays do. The dim light of dawn came into the room with a hint of reluctance, blowing the curtains on the half-open window. I sat up, alone in bed. Craig was at church. I looked around. Morning. There was nothing new to be seen in the room. It was as it had been for a long time. I put on my robe and went outside to get the paper. Although it had rained the night before, the streets didn't seem as clean as they sometimes do. They were just wet.

The girls were still sleeping when Craig returned from St. Brendan's. He went up to change, and I read the paper at the kitchen table. All of a sudden there was a loud pounding on the front door. Who in the world was that at this time of morning?

I clearly remember looking at my hand as I reached for the doorknob. I like my big old peasant hands. They remind me of who I come from, Hungarian grandparents. Unlike every other woman in Larchmont Village, I've never even had a manicure. I pulled the door toward me, looked up, and saw Nick.

He was thinner than when he'd left, had a full beard and longish hair. He was wearing some kind of Indian-looking tunic and soft cotton pants. I saw that he had gotten a large red tattoo of a diamond covering the scar on his right wrist. He had a huge smile on his face.

"Hi, Mama."

The sun had come out. Nick stood there, illuminated from behind, light bouncing. Down the steps and out onto the street it was still wet, but now the road shone like metal. Slick with oil, dirty puddles looked like rainbows to the generous eye. As lovely as that was, all I saw was everything tumbling in slow motion, landing at the bottom of the snow globe.

"Nick! What are you doing here?"

So many things ran through my head all at once. He couldn't possibly have been in Olympia yesterday and seen Paul Simon. It was too far away. Did he lie about Paul Simon or about Olympia? Why did that even matter? How was he going to get to school on time in the morning?

He had a beard. That tattoo! Craig was going to flip. I did some quick driving calculations in my head and thought, *Maybe he was in San Francisco when he saw Paul Simon!* That was certainly more plausible. Plausible? That he would hallucinate Paul Simon in a bigger city? What was wrong with me? And certainly, the bigger question was the Bob Dylan thing, in any city.

This is what happens when your kid goes crazy: suddenly you are incapable of regular, rational thought. You have to develop a whole new skill of exquisitely fine parsing. Life becomes a big laundry pile to be sorted into sections. What is crazy? What is crazy with an element of reality? What is real? Which piece of insanity relates to which piece of reality? Whites or colors?

"Everything's fine, Mom," he said as he stepped into the foyer. "I just thought I'd drive down and see you guys before school started. I decided I want to sell my truck, and I can get more money for it down here. I'll sell it today and take a plane back up tonight." His eyes were pinwheels, his speech jerky.

By now the girls and Craig were in the living room.

"What are you talking about? School starts tomorrow!" I shrieked.

The whole family adjourned to the kitchen, where we tried to understand what was going on. Nick just kept saying everything was great. Craig said he knew Nick was going to screw this up. I just kept trying to figure out if there was enough time to get Nick on a plane back to Washington. Lucy and Rose were quiet. Nick announced that he was tired and needed to rest for a minute. He got a glass of water, walked into the beige room, and shut the door.

We heard a loud crash. Nick had thrown the glass through the window, shattering it. He rushed into the kitchen ranting about Craig not being his real father. He repeated the Bob Dylan theory as the girls listened, horrified. He also told us he knew he had fathered a child, one who we were hiding from him.

"I know Trevor Sheridan is my son," he roared. "Stop lying to me."

Trevor Sheridan lived around the corner and was about eight years younger than Nick—more disturbing math with which to contend as we stirred through his toxic logic stew.

Nick was sweating profusely, and his eyes were wide enough to see the whites all around. Rimmed in alabaster, the warm brown pupils darkened chillingly. Eyes that had held only goodness before now caused me to take an actual step backward.

"Okay, that is it," Craig bellowed. "You cannot come into this house, destroy things, upset your mother and your sisters, and yell these ridiculous ideas! This is not acceptable. Get out! Get out of my house right now."

I didn't know what to do. I just wanted all of this not to be happening. All the days, all the years, all the running of interference, just to get to the point at which he would go to college. My master-piece of imagined happy ending shattering right in front of me.

"Do what your father says," I said, having run out of cards to play.

We all stood there, like players in some old Western, staring at each other. I thought back on the day now so long ago, crouching outside of Kaiser with Jenny (the sweet smell of baking bread), when I couldn't summon the courage to have him committed. That day, nobody had stepped up and slapped me across the face shouting, "Wake up!" This day, someone did—Lucy.

"Wait a minute! Mom! Dad! What are you doing? You can't just throw him out of here. Something is really wrong with him. Look at him! He's your son. You need to help him." She spoke with clarity and conviction. "Mom. Dad."

"I want him out of here," Craig said. "I will not have this in my house."

I looked at Lucy. She looked at me. "He needs to go to the hospital," she said.

I was hamstrung between my allegiance to my husband and the irrefutable truth of Nick's condition.

"Come on, Nick, come, and we'll take you. They can help you," I said.

Nick refused to go. He wanted to go to Point Dume and find

Bob Dylan and get this thing straightened out once and for all. Lucy and I convinced him that we would take him there if he would just stop by Kaiser first. Off we went, leaving Craig and Rose staring at us from the kitchen.

I can only imagine what was going on in Rose's head. When I was little, I had an older cousin who would always grab me by the wrists and swing me in a big circle until I was perpendicular to the earth. Everybody would laugh, so I knew it was supposed to be fun. In actuality, it made me nauseated, and when he put me down, I had to stay perfectly still for a minute just to get my bearings. The world around me was spinning, and I was afraid to move. That is how I imagine Rose felt, standing there in the kitchen.

My fifteen-year-old daughter became my wingman at the first hospitalization of my son. She should not have had to do that. But Craig was paralyzed, Rose was just a little girl, and Nick was on fire. I think I might have died without her.

We arrived at the emergency room. I didn't know how to explain the problem. He was acting crazy. Maybe it was drugs. Yes, he'd had psychological problems in the past. Yes, he has seen a psychiatrist. He was delusional.

They put Nick in a room with a guard outside, as is standard protocol with psych cases. He was not allowed to leave until he was evaluated by a psychiatrist. We waited.

Every time I opened my mouth, I began to cry. I couldn't ask a question; I couldn't advocate for my son; I couldn't even say my name. Lucy did everything. I spent most of the time apologizing to her for what was happening. She replied with a short "Cut it out, Ma. We're a family. We take care of each other. I'm fine."

At one point, while we were waiting for the psychiatrist, I was wandering like a bomb blast victim down the hallway. A woman pushing a big, shiny cart piled with towels and supplies walked past me. I drifted away. I continued my shell-shocked meandering. A minute later a supply closet door opened, and she pulled me in.

"Sit down, honey," she said, turning over a bucket, my makeshift seat.

What was going on now? Lucy was out there wrangling the doctors and nurses, and I was sitting in a janitor's closet?

"Listen to me. I want to tell you something," she said, looking straight at me. "My husband is sick like your son. He has the same thing. It is terrible. Those doctors are bastards. They think they are gods. The nurses, they are so overworked, they can hardly help. You gotta get strong, *mija*. You are the mother. Don't let them push you around. I know you want to just cry forever, but you can't."

She put her ample arms around me and held me while I sobbed. Then she pulled away and said, "This isn't going to go away. This is it now. Don't waste time wishing it wasn't true." She held both my hands in hers for just a second and then left.

It was a big, modern hospital. It had recently been remodeled, and everything was technologically perfect. The art on the walls was interesting and edgy. The floors were of that new, fake, better-than-real wood. Down the hall, my son was tethered to a bed with a jolly guard at the door, waiting for a psychiatrist to decide whether he was nuts or not.

All around me were sick people, scared people, busy technicians, and healers. Old ladies were wailing. The man in the room adjacent to Nick moaned with a pain I can only imagine. I'm sure someone must have died that night. Blood was everywhere. It pumped through veins and arteries; it lay in smears on the floor. It ran cold. In the midst of all that, I sat alone in a closet. At the epicenter of that astounding world, salvation was found in the arms of the lady who folds the towels.

This time I did not hesitate with regard to the hold. I begged for the hold. I wanted them to take him, figure this thing out, and return him to me, healed. Lucy and I spent about four hours there. I filled out papers, signed them, and left. Nick was infuriated that we'd double-crossed him about the Point Dume trip, but he didn't seem particularly upset about staying there. They informed us that the Kaiser psychiatric facilities were all filled, so he would be farmed out to an affiliated hospital. After some discussion about whether the quality of another place would be as good as Kaiser, I just wilted, and we went home. What was the difference? By what measure would I discern quality? Was this a four-star or a three-star nuthouse? The truth was, I just wanted to get out of there and back home, which made me feel like a monster.

After a debriefing at home, Rose and I went to Safeway. It felt so good to be walking up familiar aisles, picking out healthy food for my family, pretending nothing was wrong. The soothing grocery music played as I picked up some Oreos.

"Rosie, why don't we get some of these for a treat?"

No wonder she grew up to be furious with me. I brushed everything under an exquisite, intricate carpet in my mind. She must have thought *she* was crazy.

Over by the milk products, I saw my friend Brenda with her younger daughters.

"Hi, Mimi. How's it going?" she asked.

"I just had Nick committed to an insane asylum, and now I'm grocery shopping."

I suppose that was a way of forcing myself to accept it, but it sure wasn't a nice thing to do to Brenda. She was speechless. We had a hushed conversation. I don't know who I was hiding from, the kids or the other shoppers. Brenda was lovely; she listened and sympathized. I went home and cooked spaghetti and meatballs, Tuscany style.

Later that evening, Nick was transferred to a small hospital. First thing the next morning, Craig and I drove out there. It seemed nice, a very parklike setting. No armed guards. Maybe this wasn't so bad. Maybe they would know what to do. We were introduced to a Dr. Karamizios, who explained that Nick was on a seventy-two-hour hold, during which time they would observe and evaluate him and work toward stabilizing him on medication, and then he could be released. If they were not able to achieve this, then they would extend the hold.

We asked a lot of questions. I tried to give the doctor Nick's entire life history, but he didn't appear to consider that germane at all. This was my first glimpse of the "stabilize 'em and discharge 'em" doctrine of the mental health system. The object is to render them temporarily harmless (usually with drugs) and spit them back out into the world.

We walked down a long hall with several automatic doors before we entered the visiting room. Nick was sitting contentedly in a chair, smiling. Craig went over the details the doctor had given us and asked Nick what he thought about what was going on.

Nick tipped back in his chair, lifted his foot up for us to see, and grinned.

"Look. They took away my shoelaces."

I suppose most people would be horrified at the implications of this. For some reason we all started laughing. When sorrow is the underbelly, laughter can be the smooth, glistening pelt above.

"I guess they thought I'd hang myself," said Nick.

Gallows humor was all we had. Subjects that should be taboo for comedy were increasingly the only subjects we had. So we laughed.

We left, telling him that he had to work with the doctors and figure out what was going on. I returned the next day, and he seemed much better. The drugs were beginning to kick in, and his sentences made sense. On the third day, Craig and I arrived to hear that Nick was now stable and they were compelled by law to release him. His diagnosis of bipolar might be correct, but it was strongly recommended that he have further treatment and assessment. They gave him a prescription for an antipsychotic drug and wished us well.

As we walked out of the hospital, I said, for no reason that can ever be explained, "Wait, let's get a picture!"

A passerby took the photo of the three of us in front of the entrance of College Hospital in Cerritos. Nick stood in the middle, and we put our arms around him. Smiled. I don't know where that photo is today, but it definitely belongs in the Smithsonian, Bad Ideas Wing.

"Okay, buddy, we need to sit down and make some decisions here," Craig said.

We tried so hard to make him understand that he was sick.

"Nick, it's nothing to be ashamed of. It's a chemical imbalance. It can be corrected."

"If you had diabetes, you'd take insulin. This is the same thing."

We promised to contact Evergreen and postpone his college a semester, find the best psychiatric care available, and get him on the right medication. When all that was done, he'd return to school.

"No," he said. "I'm fine now. I want to go back up to Washington and start school."

It went back and forth for quite a while, but he was almost twenty, and it was his decision.

"Nick," I said, "I want to make this very, very clear to you. Dad and I do not support this decision. We think it is a terrible idea. If you insist on pursuing this path, you are on your own. Your tuition is paid, but you'll have to get a job."

"It's fine, Ma. I get it. Trust me, I'm going to make this work. You'll be so proud of me."

"Nick, if you disregard our wishes, you cannot return to live at the house. You will have to make your own way from here on out. Are you ready for that?" I asked, hoping desperately to scare him into staying in Los Angeles.

The midday sun beat down on our car as we zoomed toward the airport. In Los Angeles, one usually doesn't zoom anywhere, but just on the one day I wanted time to stand still, the roads were wide open. The three of us chatted inanely in the car, discussing Nick's plans, how he was going to succeed at school. I smiled at the lady in the car next to us. A bird flew into the clouds. We pulled up to the white zone to unload our disintegrating son. We hugged him. We told him we loved him.

Craig and I went to the movies. It was the middle of the day, in the middle of the week, and we went to the movies. We didn't know what else to do.

Nick lasted about seven days at Evergreen. I don't suppose I will ever know what happened up there. Somehow, he managed to drop out in time to get his tuition back, then hopped on a train headed to LA.

I don't know what happened to all the possessions he'd crammed into his truck when he first left LA. I have an image of his belongings scattered along roadside train tracks all up and down the West Coast. Oh look, there's the photo album Lucy and I made for him, so he wouldn't be lonely. It's nestled under a tree branch in Chehalis. What's that? His high school yearbook on a rock by the Cowlitz River. How in the world did his wristwatch end up on that woman outside the train station in Portland? When Nick returned on the train, all he had was a duffel bag and a box.

Craig and I were determined to stick to our edict about not letting Nick back in the house. There was no way for anyone to pretend this was normal anymore, so we waited with equal parts fear and love pounding.

On the morning of Nick's twentieth birthday, I headed toward work. He hadn't shown up in LA yet, and I figured business as usual was the way to go. I stopped at the car wash on my way there and was sitting in line when my phone rang. It was Nick's ringtone.

"Hello?" I said, rather tentatively.

"Hello," came a woman's voice. "I'm in the train station in Washington, and I found this phone, plugged in and charging. They say a young man ran to get back on the train and left it."

"How did you know to call me?" I asked.

"Oh, I just scrolled down his contacts and found 'Mom.' I figured that was who would be most worried."

"Oh, thank you so much," I said.

We chatted briefly, haltingly. She said she would send the phone to our house. I assured her that I would pay for the postage and insisted she give me her address. She said it wasn't necessary.

"I'm a mother, dear. I know how it is," she said so warmly I wanted to die.

"I don't know what to do," I said to the total stranger. "I don't know how to help him." She was very sweet but had nothing to offer. These days I found myself asking for answers anywhere. At about this same time, while in a parking garage, I actually stood fixed and stared at one of those emergency phones with a "HELP" sign mounted above it. I fought the urge to run over, pick it up, and ask, "Please. Please. What do I do about my son?"

The next day he arrived in LA. We let him leave his things on the porch but sent him away. He simply had to find another place to live. He went to stay with his friend Jack, back on Ridgewood Place, temporarily. The same friend he had been playing with, so long ago, when he asked me about the shadows. The two boys who had toddled together and later strolled and rode bikes up and down that sidewalk and street. They were now men.

Nick had some money from his tuition refund. After a few weeks, he managed to get himself into an apartment in the neighborhood. He worked intermittently at odd jobs—yard work, house painting—and seemed to function fairly well for a while. He stopped his medication, said he wanted to try on his own. He was twenty now, and I couldn't force him. Did I still think the crazy would just go away?

We had seductive conversations where he would say what I wanted to hear. They fueled my refusal to believe what was right in front of me.

"Ma, I haven't given up on going back to school. I called my counselor yesterday."

"You did?"

"Yeah. He said it would be hard, but if I pulled it together, got a note from my doctor about the medication, he'd see what he could do."

"But are you taking the medication regularly?"

"I'm going to start. You'll see. You're going to be so happy."

And I hung my hopes on that.

5

THE CRAZY DOES
NOT GO AWAY

During the months after the college debacle, things actually did settle down a bit. It was relatively peaceful at home. Scarlett came for a visit with the newest baby. Nick would come and go. He seemed to be cobbling together some kind of life. He wasn't delusional anymore, but he definitely was manic. Obsessed with "getting in shape," he could be seen jogging around the neighborhood regularly in a pair of swimming trunks covered in tiny skulls. He got very thin. He was spending time with friends, and I chose to see that as a positive sign.

Nick put a lot of effort into "creating" his apartment. He was planning on installing platforms as he had seen Kramer do in an old *Seinfeld* episode. I took him downtown to the garment district to buy fabric for his installations.

"Mama, look at this snazzy design. Do you like it?"

"That's really cool, but are you sure you should be using your money for this?"

"It's very important for an artist to have the perfect environment to create. You know that."

Nick's paintings had been precisely realistic since he was small. By the time he was in high school, his childhood drawings of farms and animals had given way to accomplished still life paintings. He was one of twelve high schoolers chosen to attend a special program at USC where they drew from live models. His figures had solidity and purpose. Now he was moving into a hybrid of recognizable images and wildly abstract visions, his colors exuberant and bold. It was exciting to watch.

We continued to nag him about the medication. He refused. He was running out of money. Craig and I agreed we would not give him any, hoping that AA's "rock bottom" theory might work.

"Mom, I don't have any food. I'm hungry. Please."

I pulled up to his apartment, leaned over to the window of the passenger side, and handed him a bag of sandwiches. Looking at him, I felt an unbearable wave of tenderness. His pale skin, the bones on his chest, his thin calves.

My son. My boy. Oh God, how did this happen? His soft hair against the side of his face was the saddest thing I had seen in my whole life. I wanted to comfort him, to hold him and save him and bring him back to our world. But he didn't like to be touched anymore. Then I said something he didn't like, and he gave me the crazy eyes. Boom. All I could do was drive away.

A week later he bounded up to the car. "Ma, I have an idea. I'm going to call the doctor to make an appointment and try the medication! I just need you to give me some money so I can do my laundry."

"No, Nick. I'm not falling for that one again. If you want clean clothes, give me your laundry, and I'll do it."

He looked at me, and I looked at him, and out of nowhere he said, "This isn't how we planned it when I was a little baby, Mom."

No shit.

At sixteen, Nick had been invited to New York for a week to work on a mural project a friend of his was doing for a women's shelter. His artistic talent and the girl's fervent crush combined to convince her parents to pay for the trip. Craig and I were sitting at a sidewalk café in Hollywood, eating breakfast, when he called.

"Let me talk to Dad, please. Let me talk to Dad."

"Oh, I'm fine, Nick. How are you?" I said.

"Ma, I'm sorry, I just need to tell him something."

I handed the phone to Craig. He listened for a while, and then his eyes welled up. "That's understandable, son. I've felt the same way. It's Picasso." He said, "Goodbye, I love you," and closed the phone.

"What?" I demanded.

As I finished my eggs Benedict, my husband relayed the story of our son, alone at the Museum of Modern Art, encountering the epic condemnation of war that is the painting *Guernica*. He had been so moved he started to cry, and that scared him. He wanted to confirm with Craig that it wasn't strange to cry while looking at art.

I drove by Nick's apartment every night to make sure a light had been turned on, so I'd know he hadn't died during the day. His behavior became erratic. He was prone to outbursts of anger. He lost contact with his friends. He was hostile to the family, me in particular. The delusions returned in full force. We were now soaring past the "Bob Dylan is my dad" galaxy.

"I know what you do, Mom. I know."

"What are you talking about?" I asked hesitantly.

"I know you're a tweaker. You're a tweaker, and you drive around all day talking with the Mexicans on your cell phone. Planning things. Talking about me."

Who was this person? It was becoming clear to me that this was moving beyond the diagnosis of bipolar, these were the "disordered thoughts" that pointed to schizophrenia. "That isn't true, Nick," I said as evenly as I could.

"And don't think I've forgotten about my baby. Trevor. I know I am his father. You can only hide all this for so long."

I bought every book about mental illness I could find. Dr. Hamill had finished his residency and moved on, so we were back at Kaiser. The psychiatric department was woefully inadequate. They allowed a fixed number of visits with a therapist per year, and if that didn't fix you, well, too bad. The tedious untangling of people's afflicted minds is not a profitable endeavor. The doctor Nick saw was not helpful. I'd had a few tantrums over there, and after that she used the privacy laws to keep me out of her office. I realized Kaiser wasn't going to save him and started reading.

Craig asked me, "Does this ever just go away? Do people with mental illness ever really get better?"

"Well," I said, "approximately one percent of the population gets schizophrenia. Of those people, there is a genetic component that increases with the number of afflicted family members. But the majority of the one percent is not genetically related. Ten years after initial diagnosis, approximately twenty-five percent of people diagnosed with schizophrenia recover."

"Been doing some reading, huh?" he asked.

"I don't know what else to do. He sure seems to meet the criteria for schizophrenia. Maybe he'll be in the group where it runs its course in ten years."

"Let's talk about something else, Dr. Feldman."

This was the beginning of a pattern in our relationship that would last for many years. At the bedrock of our marriage—glittering slightly even in the dark, more profound than our tether to artmaking—was the fact that we had made children together. Human beings. While that bound us permanently, it also separated us. When we discussed his illness, our combined misery grew exponentially to the point where it was unbearable. We stopped talking about Nick unless it was of a practical nature. I did a lot of solitary crying. I drank a lot. Recently, I asked Craig what he was doing during that time to cope. Did he also pull to the side of some shady, treelined street and sob his eyes out? Did he realize he retreated from all of us, disappeared? He said he did. Do I know the arithmetic of his guilt and regret? No. I only know my own.

Nick and I were sitting in our favorite Lebanese restaurant. On the table before us lay an array of Middle Eastern delights: hummus, eggplant, tahini, my favorite cucumber and tomato salad. He was telling me all about the Illuminati. I sat there, numb, as it all filtered in.

"I'm really not sure what that is, Nick. It sounds a little out there to me," I said, trying to keep just one foot in the real world.

"How can you say that, Mom? You were the one who taught me about all this."

"What are you talking about? I taught you what?"

"Remember when I was little and you told me about the government? About how they can hear us and see us and all that?"

Oh boy.

"Nick, you're scaring me. I don't know what you mean."

"It's the televisions. And the cameras. And only the Illuminati know the truth."

The hummus turned to chalk in my mouth. The restaurant noise faded, and my face grew hot.

As the days went by, I noticed more changes. His paranoia and delusions became fairly constant; his speech patterns changed entirely. Where once he spoke coherently about deranged ideas, now the actual speech itself was distorted. He was using made-up words all the time.

"I've been reading Bukowski, Ma, and I'm concerned about his reprement."

"His what?" I asked quietly.

"Repremention! It's upsetting."

"Oh, I wouldn't worry too much about that, Nicknack. Why don't you switch back to Salinger?" I suggested.

"Them!" He perked up.

"Them?"

"You know, *Franny and Zooey*, the *original* Salinger. Not that bigheaded monkey."

I looked at him. He returned my bewilderment with one of his blinding, life-altering smiles. "You know, the old Salinger, not the new stuff."

He had a great deal of difficulty focusing and responding to others. It began at last to dawn on me—Nick really was hearing voices in his head and responding to them out loud.

As Nick let go of reality, I couldn't help but note that he was doing it in a very interesting way. When I was able to pull back, I would think, *Hmm. He's really brilliant.* What, exactly, is the delineation between brilliance and lunacy? Is there one?

He began to harass people unknowingly, trying to be friendly. He became fixated on a woman who lived in his building. We were told by the building manager that he screamed and yelled when he was alone in his apartment. An old friend of his called me because she had visited and found his bathtub filled to the rim with salsa. Interesting? Not so much.

I knew his savings were diminishing. What does a bathtub full of salsa cost?

One day I summoned all my courage and went over there with my friend Brooke. We furtively slid down the hallways, up the stairways, ready for anything. We ended up pounding on his apartment door for ten minutes and then just leaving because I didn't know what else to do. I could have pounded forever.

A friend told me about the National Alliance on Mental Illness, an advocacy group. NAMI has a twelve-week educational program called Family-to-Family, which I certainly needed. The first night I went, we weren't five minutes in when my phone rang.

"Mama, Mama, all the lights are out. We're scared!" It was Lucy. I could hear Rose whimpering.

"Calm down, Lulu." My teeth hurt. "There's probably just a power outage. Go look out the front window and tell me if other lights are on."

"They are, Mom! It's only our house. What's going on?"

"Okay. This is what I want you to do. Take Rose and go over to Theresa's house. Just shut the door behind you, and go across the street. I'll call T and tell her you're coming."

I returned to the house to find someone had flipped all the breaker switches in the outside box. Someone. Taped to the box was this note:

> To the parking attendants in Los Angeles:
> Listen closely
> Listen deeply
> Look deeply into yourself and think about your joys,
> happiness and integrity.
> Now listen here please . . .
> Give up your profession,
> throw down those god-awful new computerized ticket thingies.
> Break 'em!
> I will pay you from here on out to write sorry notes/love letters
> to any person who has received a parking ticket,
> and you are all invited to my annual Christmas Party/Hanukkah
>   Celebration.

I didn't bother asking him about it. I just bought a padlock and put it on the breaker box. I called Craig in Washington and told him it was time to come home.

"Why, what's going on?" he asked.

I relayed the whole episode in exacting detail.

"I don't even know who he is anymore."

"Join the club," I said.

"I'll be there as soon as I can."

That night, after the girls went to bed, I watched some old family videos. I needed to remember that it hadn't always been like this. After a few birthday parties, I slipped in a tape labeled "Road Trip

2001," which I had never seen before.

Fifteen-year-old Nick is holding the camera. We see Craig's profile against the geometry of the driver's window, nodding. He waves out the window to the flatlands of Utah. Bob Dylan is playing indistinctly, goats line the side of the road, tumbling winds sound, like a movie. The camera holds for a moment on Craig against the red rocks, the orange rocks. He's wearing a cap and a purple shirt.

"Dad, where are we?"

"We just crossed Monument Valley," Craig says to Nick. Then, to the world at large: "June twenty-third, two thousand and one. On our way to Colorado. Uncle Cal's funeral."

Nick, breathy, "Look at the clouds!"

Craig, deeply, "God rest his soul."

Handing out free tickets to the wedding of his son . . . Bob. Different road now, greener land, a truck whizzes by, and they sing together . . . *to get caught without a ticket and be discovered . . .* A huge silver truck is a rectangle in front of them. Bob whines . . . *and it strangled up my mind . . .* indistinct talking between Craig and Nick . . . *oh, Mama, can this really be the end, to be stuck inside of Mobile with the Memphis blues again . . .*

Cut to different scenery. Nick emits a boyish screech and then "Aughhhh!" as he moves the lens across blue beveled valleys . . . *all I reaaaallly want to doooo, is, baby, be friends with you . . .*

Now water splashing on the windshield, slapping wipers remove dirt, Nick's teenage voice lilts with happiness, "So great. We haven't been in so long." Snaking water in streams all around the rocky land . . . *I was so much older then, I'm younger than that now . . .* The camera moves to reveal Craig's face as they pull into a funky little motel. A truck is parked, and as Craig pulls up next to it, he says softly, "Oh, look at that old Land Cruiser. Don't you love them?"

"I love them," Nick says.

Now wind, wind howling loud like animals, and Craig shouts, "Like an American scene, mountain land! God's country." We hear

Nick chuckle. The gentle rhythm between a father and a son—familiar, clipped.

A close up of Nick's eye fills the whole screen. Then nose, nostrils, swooping back to the sky as Bob sings . . . *but I was so much older then, I'm younger than that now* . . . Someone burps loudly, and they both laugh. "We're back!" Craig's voice booms as we see the "Welcome to Colorado" sign.

"Clouds in Colorado!" Nick bellows. "Bob Dylan in Colorado!" They both start to sing along to the music . . . *true love, true love, true love tends to forget* . . . Flying by an old mill, tall grass, Nick zooms in on a cow.

Craig has the camera now. Nick stands near him by the side of the road in a bright-blue hoodie, smiling vaguely. Oh, he is so tall and muscular and handsome. He walks with all the assurance of adolescence. No words are spoken as Nick heads out into the hills. Craig watches him, through the lens, getting smaller and smaller. He starts running, arms waving, childlike, and then he stops and looks back at his father. "God's country!" he laughs.

Wipers tick back and forth, glinting snow in the distance; a whole story is sketched across the windshield in watery script. "Look, it's a school bus, Nick." Then quiet but for the harmonica on the car radio.

Nick is standing on a ridge in silly plastic sandals and shorts. The sign says Cottonwood Pass. He beams a giant smile at his dad and says, "Isn't this fucking amazing?" Craig keeps the camera on Nick as he meanders. It's getting darker now, and the brown clouds are reflected in the lake.

Bright view of a large white farmhouse and the verdant land surrounding Craig's grandfather's ranch, which was lost years ago to back taxes and debt. "I want to get a picture of you and the ranch." The camera moves from the corral back to the car. "I want you to get the ranch back, Nick." Nick smiles and lackadaisically points a finger out the window toward the house.

"Why don't you make that your life's mission?" Craig flicks a bug off his arm. "What do you say about that?"

Nick nods in a manly way, his T-shirt sparkling white, and says softly, "I'm gonna get it back."

Driving down a two-lane blacktop, Nick's voice rings out, "Leadville, Colorado!" Craggy gold-green earth, and cars dotting the hills. Craig begins making banjo sounds. "Yeehaaaw!" Nick yells as Bob croons . . . *but, oh, what a wonderful feeling* . . . and they head down a dirt road past two rusted trailers nestled together like an old couple. No talk, just a father and son looking at cars, fences, and junk. *New Morning* plays on the radio.

They are out of the car, standing on some railroad tracks. Behind them is a tent and smoldering campfire. The camera moves to the left, where rain clouds darken a couple of grazing horses, and we hear Nick say "Ahhhh." The camera follows some electrical lines as Nick makes guitar noises. Suddenly the camera is close on Craig making a face and grunting "Yeah!" Nick says, affectionately, "Look at this guy." Craig mugs for the camera, making more faces, smiling like a kid.

Nick, behind the camera, murmurs, "What a crazy fool," in the most melodic and loving voice ever spoken on this earth.

During the week Craig was locking up in Washington, Nick attempted to break into his neighbor's apartment in the middle of the night. Twice. She called the landlord, who called the police. Nick was evicted. He had three days to get out.

"What do we do now? I don't know what to do now!"

"You cannot let him back into the house, Mimi," Craig said.

"I know. We have to keep him away from the girls. After the breaker-box thing, they're really nervous."

"You talked to the management company?"

"They wouldn't even discuss it. If he isn't out by Tuesday, the police will be called and charges filed."

"What kind of outfit is this management company? They can't just do that!"

"Evidently, they can. Imagine how scared the woman must be."

We talked for about an hour. We couldn't let him move home, and he wouldn't go to a hospital. He was going to end up homeless. Should we call a lawyer? It went on and on with no resolution.

Suddenly Craig said loudly, "Mimi! This is really bad. Don't you know having an eviction on your record seriously screws up your credit rating?"

His credit rating?

"I think Nick's *credit rating* is pretty low down on the list of his problems right now. You better load up that truck and hit the road fast, man. It's getting bad down here."

Nick managed to finagle his way back into Jack's garage (Bridget was afraid to have him in the house by then). He was back on Ridgewood Place, three doors from our old house.

Nick showed up on the front porch the night before Craig got home.

"I just want to come in and visit," he said.

"Nick, you have to leave. I told you that you can't be here."

"C'mon, Mom, I just want something to eat. What's the big deal?"

I told him that if he didn't leave, I would call the police. He was trespassing. I had learned that these situations can be an opportunity. If you call the police, there is the possibility that you can get them hospitalized. There is also the possibility that someone could end up dead; you read of police shootings like that all the time. Loved ones call for help because a person is sick, and the police, feeling threatened, shoot. Some of the larger cities have special training for officers in dealing with mental health cases, but most do not. The stakes are high when seeking assistance, and it is small wonder so many people hide the truth.

Nick got angrier and angrier. The girls ran upstairs. He pounded on the door. I called the damn police. They took Nick down to the sidewalk and spoke with him privately. He managed to convince them that he was fine and agreed to leave. I know now that I should have lied and said he was threatening suicide or cited one of the other very narrow guidelines that require them to take him. That night I just stood with my back to the street, looking at my daughters.

"If you let him move back in here, we are moving out." Lucy stood slightly in front of Rose, her long, unkempt hair the perfect foil to Rose's straight brown mane. Two child warriors.

The next morning, I drove to the police station. I was in my work clothes, so I fit in well with the crowd down there. Uncombed hair, covered in paint, and borderline hysterical, I tried to distinguish myself from the crackheads, the homeless, and the petty criminals. After all, I was an upright citizen who needed help.

"Excuse me, sir, but I have a very serious situation with my son that needs attending to," I said in my most authoritative voice.

They listened and then explained why there was nothing they could do. I had to wait until something actually happened. A crime, or the attempt at one. So . . . if Nick would just stab someone, we'd be in business.

I have thrown myself at the mercy of policemen, doctors, mental health practitioners, and social workers with an abandonment of pride I never thought I'd allow, and repeatedly, there is nothing that any of them can do. How could this be, in the modern world? I began to be driven by anger mixed with fear.

When Craig returned, we tried to get through to Nick, but he had no awareness about his illness. There is a word for that: *anosognosia*. The real or feigned ignorance of the presence of a disease. It makes sense; the very organ that is sick is the one that would allow you to understand that you are sick.

His behavior was becoming completely uncontrolled. He came to the house and yelled on the front lawn. He hid in the bushes and only left at the threat of police. At my wit's end, I wrote a letter, hoping that paper would somehow give our message more power. I told him he was legally forbidden on our property, attaching a long list of family, friends, doctors, and help lines. I offered to help if he would go on medication. I handed it to Craig, and he signed his name next to mine. I cannot calculate what banning my own son from his home cost my soul, but I had to protect the girls. This disease may have had its hand on Nick, but I was going to win. In the meantime, I sure as hell wasn't going to allow it to destroy my family.

I handed the letter to dear Bridget and asked her to pass it on, apologizing about a hundred times. We both knew it was dangerous for her to have Nick there. I thought of that rainy day I had picked up my small boy from her house. The day little crystal droplets of rain had kissed the leaves and we'd talked about shadows. The longing for that time was like a sharp wire around my belly.

Afterward, I sat in the car for a while, unable to move. I thought, *I am sick of being strong. My skills are no match for this. Either let me save him or let me lie down and die. This is happening because I can't figure out what to do. I call and I read and I talk. I do research. I turn to friends. I go to people smarter than me. I go to ghosts and I yell at God, but I can't find anyone to tell me what to do. There is no map. Everybody sympathizes and empathizes and shakes their head. But there is no map. GIVE ME THE MOTHERFUCKING MAP.*

I couldn't just sit in the car forever, feeling sorry for myself. After all, Rose had a dentist appointment.

I went to the second NAMI meeting. I had to acquire some skills for coping. Craig would do what I asked of him, but he was disappearing as things got worse. Nick was roaming the neighborhood, sleeping in Jack's garage, hanging out with some pretty shady characters. Things were bad.

The NAMI program was excellent. It was divided into twelve sessions, each one tackling one aspect of mental illness. It included things like the science of mental illnesses, the health system, different medications, law enforcement, and treatment options. Finally, something tangible.

We all introduced ourselves. There were several couples, some single mothers, siblings. We came to a young woman with bright eyes and tapered fingernails painted pink.

"Hi, I'm LaTonya," she said. "My boyfriend has schizophrenia. We've been together for a year. I truly love him and want to make this work."

I looked at that smooth young face, and I wanted to yell, "Run! Run now! As far and as fast as you can!"

Back at the table, the parents seemed mostly conflicted, or clearly one had dragged the other in. Everybody was sad, scared, and tired. When it was my turn to speak, I said, "Hi, I'm Mimi. My son, Nick, is . . . has . . . is nuts."

You could have heard a pin drop.

I was politely informed that it is politically incorrect to use the term "nuts." The leader took the opportunity to talk about stigma. She passed around a copy of a cartoon that had appeared in a magazine. It depicted a courtroom and a defendant with the traditional tinfoil hat that is code for insanity. I had such a desperate need to find some humor in my life that I actually laughed—the rest of them stared at me with disdain.

Stigma. It might be the biggest impediment to the early and accurate diagnosis of mental illness, worse than the science of the disease, worse than the manifestations. It multiplies the suffering. The fear of stigma prevents people from seeking treatment. People with cancer don't typically feel shame. Mental illness has such a long history of misconceptions and discrimination. No one wants to talk about it. We shove it into corners; we hide Auntie in the attic; we find other less formidable names for it that serve to trivialize it as "a bit ditzy" or "cuckoo." We look away from the guy screaming on the corner.

Now the guy on the corner is my own son.

There is virtually no functioning mental health system in America. The majority of the mentally ill are either homeless or in jails, which have become our de facto psychiatric facilities. I began to see that the hamster wheel I had been on for the past few years was not of my own making. It was simply how this worked.

Stigma. I had gotten over stigma a long time ago. The first night I had police on my porch and saw the neighbors' horrified, judgy faces, I suspected even then that it was pointless to care. Actually, one of the perks of having a son with schizophrenia is that you become officially embarrassment-proof. *Let them stare. I've got a job to do.*

When Rose was about twelve, she used to do a comical impersonation of me.

"Look. This is Mom." She'd pick up the phone and in her most ripened, singsongy voice, mimic me: "Hello, my name is Miriam Feldman, and I have a son with schizophrenia. I'm wondering if you can help me . . ." It was good.

I do it on purpose. I say the words. I don't hide. It is bad enough that my son has this terrible disease. I'm supposed to be ashamed too? It is not incumbent upon me to shield others from the ugliness of mental illness. It is the most compelling duty of humanity that we *all* look it in the eye.

At the next meeting, I decided to be a little more low-key. I wasn't making any friends around there. The subject was understanding how the different illnesses felt. We did an exercise on schizophrenia. Half of us sat around the table with a paper and pencil, one person standing behind each of us. The leader was in front with a dry-erase board.

Each standing person was given a piece of paper with a narrative that went something like this: "Do not listen to the person directing you. They are the devil. They are trying to trick you. They want to hurt you." Each script was different, but the message was the same. The exercise required the person sitting to follow a simple sequence of visual directions to create a design on our paper. The leader would tell the sitting person to draw a one-inch vertical line, then a circle. While she was giving directions, the person standing was to bend over and speak his or her script into the ear of the sitter.

I sat at the table, trying to draw the circle, while a large man stood behind me and warned repeatedly that someone was going to mutilate and kill me. In addition to that, the noise from all the talkers made it almost impossible to hear the leader. It was like the cacophony of a school recess yard—uncontrollable, barbarian, indecipherable.

The leader called out, "Okay, stop now!" It took a while to wind down. The tension in that room was overwhelming. As it finally fell quiet, the leader softly said, "That is what it is like for your loved one with schizophrenia every minute of every day." She explained the neurological workings that eliminated the filter we all have to prioritize sounds. A normal brain is able to pay primary attention to one thing, while still being aware of ambient noise. To the schizophrenic brain, it all comes in, full speed ahead, and added to that are auditory hallucinations. They don't know which direction to turn.

After the exercise, we did some sharing. The very sweet couple next to me recounted the circumstances of the past week. Their forty-seven-year-old son was still living on their condominium balcony, under a wrought iron decorative table they bought to sit at and enjoy their morning coffee. It had been three years, and he showed no signs of leaving.

LaTonya was still hanging in there with the boyfriend. He was getting violent and had started throwing things. In the middle of the night, he'd wake up screaming. Once awake, it didn't stop because it wasn't a dream, it was the madness. Every week I fought the impulse to take her aside and tell her to get out of the relationship.

David, the overweight IT guy, whose mother *and* sister have schizophrenia, was a little depressed that week. *That week?* My sense of humor had begun to wane. I looked at the sad, faded blue shirt that matched his eyes and imagined what it would be like to be him. You couldn't even consider having children because of the genetics, and what woman would sign up for that (aside from LaTonya)?

All he does is go to work and then try to control the damage. Every day.

The door opened, and a woman peeked in. Behind her was her son. He was large, scrubbed, and nicely dressed. She was small, round, and precisely made-up. It was clearly the big day: she had gotten him to come. She was nothing like me. She was wearing a suit and pearls and had a hairdo. I was crouched in my chair, wearing jeans and sporting messy, paint-spattered hair. But I knew her all right, I sure did. She was *exactly* like me.

That same hopeful expression—was this going to be the place that improved things? That ridiculous "putting a good face on it" determination. This mother, holding the pieces of her broken heart in her own hands. An organ busted so recklessly, so raggedly, that the shards, in turn, cut *her*. The very hands that were holding it together.

Oh, I know her.

Walking to my car after the meeting, I couldn't remember what there ever was in the entire world to be amused by. I felt myself harden against the sorrow welling up inside. The sharp little tip of the car door licked the skin of my cheek as I yanked it open. That tiny prick of pain was enough. It tore me apart. I sat in the car and railed at the night sky.

"Where are you? What are you doing while my son is going mad? Where is my mother? Where is my father? Fuck you. Fuck you and the big fat faith all you believers cling to. If it's true, then where the hell are you?" I screamed. "Where are you?"

I wiped my cheek with the back of my hand, saw a faint line of blood.

"My mother told me that my hands were touched by you, that was why I could paint. I go into the colors and the movement and there I know myself, and there I lose myself. And then there I find myself. So thanks for that—the painting thing. But how about I give that back to you and you give Nick back to me? I'll never paint again. Just please, please give me back my son."

The previous week's meeting had been all about violence and the horrible things that mentally ill people sometimes do to others.

The data shows that quite often "others" means Mom. I now understand those women who go foolishly into situations of grave danger because they trust their child will know them and would never hurt them. You see it on the news all the time.

She thinks, *He'll come to his senses. He will look into my eyes, and he will stop.* We don't believe they will ever harm us, and then out comes the gun, the knife, the icy clench of strong fingers around a throat, and it is too late.

6

IT'S NOT WORTH
THE CEREAL

Nick stayed away from the house. Lucy and Rose relaxed a bit, feeling safe again. The early spring days were lengthening; you could hear kids playing outside after dinner. I was washing up so the girls could get to their homework. The kitchen TV was on, some game show, and I cleared the food from the table. I liked that time of day, when domestic chores reaffirmed some standard of normalcy.

It was getting late, and there were things to do upstairs. I turned off the TV and switched off the lights. With the house dark, the yard became more visible. I could see the maple tree against the almost-night sky. The large windows of Craig's woodshop reflected the lights in Lucy's room. At the entrance to the secret garden, there is a river rock wall Craig and the kids built together. Near the wall is an arbor of climbing roses. Under its arch stood Nick, arms at his sides, watching the activities in his now off-limits home. I pretended I didn't see him. I couldn't bear having to tell him to leave.

When Nick was still inside of me, almost born, he'd sometimes get still for a while, and then I'd worry. I could grab the heel of his foot, just below my rib, and shake it back and forth. He'd wake up, move, and I'd know he was okay. There was no heel to grab this night. He was sealed away from me on the other side of the window.

My friend Laura is a counselor at a mental health facility. One night in her living room over red wine, she said, "You know, Mimi, you absolutely should get Nick onto SSI and Medi-Cal."

"Why?" I asked. "He's on our Kaiser."

"Well, he can't stay on your coverage forever, and the medications can get very expensive. Without coverage, hospitalizations can cost tens of thousands."

Wait a minute, I thought. *She's talking like this is going to go on forever.*

"What exactly is SSI?" I asked.

"It's disability," Laura said. "Supplemental Security Income. It's really hard to get. You should start right away. He'll need permanent disability."

Wait. What? *Permanent* disability? He's going to get better when we get him on the meds. He'll have a regular life. Anyway, we can take care of our own son.

"Is that medical coverage, or do they get money too?"

"Oh, yeah, they get about eight hundred a month. It's not a lot, but it's something."

Laura explained the complicated process. I poured more wine.

When I told Craig, his reaction was similar to mine. The very idea was another move toward admitting the truth: Nick wasn't getting better. Also, it felt like charity.

"I mean, we could use the money, but I just feel like it would be wrong somehow. It would be like being on the dole. We aren't *those people*."

"I know," I said, "but we weren't *those people* who had a son who was mentally ill either. And now we are."

"Let's just think about it for a while." Craig's favorite approach.

We thought. Having a son with schizophrenia did not embarrass me, but somehow this did. Public assistance? It felt like we were scamming the system. I'd worked hard to build my painting business, compromised many of my heady ideas about art, and we got by. We weren't rich, but we weren't poor. I looked at the costs of his medications. I dug out the bill from College Hospital (that Kaiser had covered), and it was $17,000. I realized that we very well could end up poor.

"I think we should apply for the SSI," I told my husband. "I've gone over and over this, and I think we'd be stupid not to."

"I guess so. It just feels so wrong somehow."

"Hey, look at it this way," I said. "He *is* sick. This is real. This is what the system is set up for. We've been paying into it all our lives."

"I know," Craig mumbled. "I just hate this. I hate it."

"I hate everyone," I said. "And everything."

Back then, I'd keep it together during the day and then drink and cry in the bathroom at night with the shower on. It worked pretty well. The more I took on, the more Craig relinquished. One night I emerged from a sob-fest to find Lucy standing there.

"Mommy, what's wrong? You're crying."

I couldn't fake it. "I'm crying because I miss your brother, Lu."

"What do you mean, you miss him? He's not gone. He's still here," she said.

"I know," I said, "but he's not who he was supposed to be."

She looked at me plaintively and said, "Yes, he is. It's just not what *you* thought."

I went into my studio and poured myself another glass of wine. I knew my drinking was getting out of hand, and that worried me. Alcohol had almost ended my marriage. Craig is sober, had been for a dozen years at that point, but the fear never fully goes away. For years I had treaded lightly through my days, afraid of the next blowup. When Rose was an infant, I finally left. Drove right over the lawn into the street, with three kids, because Craig's car was blocking mine in the driveway. He stood yelling at me from the front porch. Faced with losing everything, he actually stopped drinking. Looking at my glass, I wondered where I was heading.

The decision to pursue the SSI allowed for a more realistic approach in dealing with the Nick Situation.

The first order of business was to find him a place to live. My bright idea was to try and get him into a sober living house. I figured we could just leave out the being mentally ill part and slide him right on in there. If he had a roof over his head and three squares, in addition to being prohibited from doing drugs, well, we'd be ahead of the game.

Nick made himself as presentable as possible. He knew he had to find a place to live. Even in his deteriorating condition, he knew that he did not want to be homeless. With clean clothes, a shave, and a haircut he looked terrific. He was still so handsome, his face articulated by his father's bone structure—strong and thoughtful. He was tall and slim then. People's heads turned. Maybe we *could* pull this off. I tried to smooth his jacket, but he moved away from my touch. We set out to visit some potential places. We'd coached him up, told him to be polite but concise.

We pulled up to a dull stucco box of a house in one of the redundant suburbs of LA. All the windows and doors had curling metal bars, pretending to be decorative. We were greeted by Dave, who ran the place.

"We have six residents here, not counting me," he said as he showed us around, telling us the house rules. He introduced us to some guys who were smoking in the backyard.

Back in the kitchen, we filled out the application. Nick was staring intently at the wall behind the stove.

"Do you have any questions, Nick?" Dave asked.

Nick pointed to the spotless wall. "Is that a drop of red wine, or is it a ladybug?"

Dave politely showed us to the door.

After being ushered out of the third place that day, we gave up and headed home.

During this stage of Nick's insanity, he'd begun to talk to himself, scat style. The indecipherable riffing in the back seat continued intermittently as Craig and I drove silently, out of ideas.

"Hey, Dad, could you just drop me at Cactus Burrito instead of home? I'm hungry," he asked.

"Do you have any money?" Craig asked.

"Yeah, I think I do. Yeah, I do."

"Wait, I thought they said that you couldn't go there anymore?" I asked. He had been overstaying his welcome around town, making scenes. Every time he went to this restaurant, he tried to convince them to let him repaint their large mural.

"Oh, we have an understanding now," Nick said.

"An understanding?"

"Yeah, I can still go there, but I can't go there too many times."

Craig and I exchanged a glance.

After the sober living folly, we got on the computer and dug a little deeper. It turned out there were also such establishments for the mentally ill. Craig compiled a list, written in perfect small cursive on a series of Post-its, as was his custom. The first prospect was chosen by location; it was mere blocks from our house. Pulling up in front, it appeared acceptable, if a little run-down. It was one of the few single-family houses that still lined Crenshaw Boulevard, now a busy street. We were greeted by Pearl, a plump woman in her forties. As she opened the door, we were almost knocked off our feet by the smell of fried chicken.

"I would like to introduce you to Robert," Pearl said. "He is one of the residents here and will help me show you around." Robert was dressed in chinos and a short-sleeved shirt, hair combed awkwardly, his skin pale.

"Nice to meet you, Robert," Craig and I both said.

We were shown the downstairs, spare but acceptable. Several chain-smoking residents relaxed on the front porch under a "No Smoking" sign. We went upstairs to look at the bedrooms. Robert led us into his room at the front of the house. It had peeling wallpaper and water stains on the ceiling. There were clothes and shoes every-where, trash cans overflowing.

"This is the room with an available bed," Pearl said. "Robert sleeps right here."

"Oh, nice," I murmured. The chicken smell was becoming a taste. You could hear people talking to themselves in their rooms. The residents either stared with empty eyes or were desperate to strike up a conversation. I thought I saw a mouse run across the hall.

I had a primal urge to get out of there. Mercifully, Pearl decided to wrap up the tour. Once in the common room, we all ricocheted thank-yous, exchanging smiles. I knew, of course, that I would never put Nick in a place like this. One look at Craig, and I knew he agreed. He extended his hand to Robert and said, "Very nice to have met you."

Robert looked back at Craig with the most earnest face I have ever seen and said, "You're really going to like it here."

Once we were safely back in the car, I said, "You're really going to like it here," but we couldn't even laugh. The place was so awful we never even looked at another. So much for the mental health boarding facilities. It's just a racket. Someone buys an old, falling-down house, staffs it with unqualified workers, then fills it with sick people. The cost per month is—surprise—*exactly* the same as the person's disability check. It's a gold mine, if you can sleep at night.

It was early evening, and most of the houses back in our neigh-borhood had lights on. From the outside, all the people looked happy and content. I could see into one kitchen after another, rows of dinners, nutritious and good. In our car, there was quiet.

We don't belong here, I thought. *We aren't like them.*

Upstairs in my office, a pile of mail awaited. On top was a jury summons for Nick, the second one in six months. Yep, he'd make a great juror. Under that was the latest issue of *People* magazine. On the cover was a famous actress who had just gone public with the fact that she was bipolar. I devoured the article like I always do. Her husband, another famous actor, had taken her to a facility where she stayed for a couple months, and they fixed her. They cured her!

Quickly, I googled the place and pulled up its website. It was located on seven beautiful acres in Virginia. The most renowned specialists in the world treated the whole person, not just the disease. It cost $45,000 a month.

We had a decent amount of equity in our house, but this would eat that up in a matter of months. We didn't have savings or retirement accounts; we were a couple of hapless artists who had lucked into a good neighborhood. I sat with my forehead on the desk, feeling the cool wood under my skin.

The next day I told Craig about the place in Virginia. For a minute we actually considered it. But we couldn't sacrifice the girls' college and security, our retirement nest egg, on a long shot like that.

Of course, operating alone, I would have done it in a second.

Thank God I wasn't operating alone.

We had to find Nick a place to live. Bridget had finally given him a deadline: the end of the month.

"Craig, the NAMI lady said that sometimes you just have to let go, let them just go homeless, and hope that they find their way. When you've tried everything."

"You know you could never do that," he said. "Why even talk about it?"

"I know. I know." I closed my eyes hard, pushed the heels of my hands into the sockets. "Okay, I have an idea," I said. "Maybe we could solve two things here. He *has* expressed concern about being homeless. What if I go to him and tell him we will get him an apartment if he goes on the meds? The old bribing technique. It's Dr. Hamill approved."

"Oh, right. Like that's gonna work. You're dreaming."

"It's worth a try! You got any better ideas?"

A waxen quiet filled the room.

"Could we afford it?" Craig whispered.

"I think we could. You know, a single somewhere south of here. If we get the SSI, it would actually be doable."

I went to talk to Nick. I told him that if he would take medication, we would provide a roof over his head, food, and a pack of cigarettes a day. That would be the deal. I didn't have much hope as I laid out the proposition.

"Okay," Nick said. "That sounds fine."

And just like that, the clouds parted.

We found Nick a studio apartment about seven blocks away, close enough to check in on him every day but also far enough for some breathing room. There was a church right across the street, which for some reason I found comforting. The apartment had been redone— new carpet, new kitchen, new paint. He'd have a fresh start there. He'd begun the meds a few days before, and I thought I could see a difference already.

How did I make peace with sending him into the world alone? Have I no shame at my own naked relief in getting away from him? People still ask why he doesn't live with us. One might as well ask "Why don't you just build a bonfire in the middle of the living room if you are cold?" I live at the intersection of love and danger. I am afraid of my own son. Every day is a crucible.

I chipped away at the SSI process. The hoops to jump through: the forms filled out, lost, filled out again, not received, missing, lost, misfiled apparently, filled out again, and then delivered in person. The steeplechase went on for weeks. I lived on the telephone. It all came down to a meeting with a doctor at the Alpine Medical Group, a facility authorized by the government to make these decisions. Nick was to be evaluated by a doctor who had never seen him before, for fifteen minutes, and that man would have the final say.

Craig and I nervously drove to get him. Everything depended on this.

Nick was agitated. Whatever I said made it worse, so I stopped talking.

It was quite far away, and there was a lot of traffic. Nick began his riffing. There was a new side effect from the medication: tardive dyskinesia. Involuntary muscle movements. There is some controversy, because it could be part of the disease in addition to a side effect of the medication. For some people, it manifests in the tongue and mouth, chewing and sucking, smacking the lips. Occasionally it can appear as jerky movements of the arms or legs. Nick's particular version was to slam the insides of his forearms together repeatedly, his palms skyward. It was startling and scary to others. By the time Craig pulled into the parking lot, Nick was banging his arms together, and yelling at me because he didn't like the way I was breathing.

Well, at least there'll be no doubt about his condition, I thought grimly.

"Okay, Nickboy, let's go on in there," Craig said.

"No. It's not worth the cereal!"

Here we go, I thought.

"Come on," Craig said calmly. "It won't take long."

Nick yelled, "I'm not going in if *she's* with us!"

"Okay, okay. I'll just walk in with you," Craig said. "Just you and me, Bub."

As I shrunk down to my smallest self in the back seat, he managed to get Nick to go in. I skulked behind them. Nick glared at me, and I watched the cracked television mounted in the corner. Jenny Jones was discussing the challenges of African American hair with a panel of women. Craig went in to answer some preliminary questions. Nick stomped his foot.

The doctor saw Nick for quite a while. When he came out, the doctor looked at Craig and raised his eyebrows. "Don't worry," he said. "He will be approved."

We were in a new life—a life where the doctor doing the equivalent to circling his index finger round and round next to his ear was cause for celebration. Nick was approved for SSI ten days later.

Things settled down. Nick was taking his Zyprexa and gradually began to improve. The myth of full recovery abandoned, I watched him carefully. Schizophrenia creates two sets of symptoms: positive and negative. The positive symptoms are not "positive" as in "good." They are the behaviors that are added to the person, such as hearing voices, hallucinations, paranoia, and delusions. The medications available address these symptoms quite well, but not without cost.

The side effects one must contend with are awful, varying with the different medications. The negative symptoms are the elements that are lost to the person with the disease, such as the ability to feel emotions, to reason logically, to empathize. It is called the "flat affect." These symptoms are not corrected by the medication; in many cases, they're exacerbated. The drugs also change in their effectiveness over time. What worked beautifully for a while can fail after a few years.

Often, the patient will decide to stop the medication himself. Sometimes, as he begins to improve (because of the medication), he decides he's cured and stops. The side effects can feel intolerable, worse than the disease itself, and also provide a reason to quit. The doctor must continuously reevaluate and adjust the combinations and dosages. We took Nick regularly to see the psychiatrist, and she gradually increased his dosage and added other things. The positive symptoms were fading. He was more alert.

We lifted the ban on his coming to our house, and, often, he would walk up to have dinner with us. He had just turned twenty-one.

"Hey, Nickboy, you here to eat? Go up and tell the girls it's ready, okay?" I walked into the kitchen.

Lucy and Rose started arguing excitedly. Some Beatles music was playing in the background, and I almost ran up there. You never knew what could happen.

"Hey, hey," I heard him say calmly. "What are you guys doing? It's sacrilegious to argue while the Beatles are playing! That's just wrong.

Let's listen to the end of the song, and then Mom wants you to come down for dinner."

I peeked around the doorway and saw the three of them in the window seat. Nick, tall beside them. Lucy looking at him adoringly. Her hand lay on the cushion, fingers reaching in his direction. Rose sat on her hands, her cheek barely grazing Lucy's shoulder as she gazed out the window.

You never knew what could happen.

7

NOT SO FAST

I had been calling Nick all morning. The familiar drumbeat of worry was closing in, so I decided to just drive down there rather than lose another day to needless anxiety.

I rang the bell. I knocked and knocked some more. He didn't answer for a long time. Finally, disheveled, he opened the door and stood in front of me, spectral and wobbly. His mouth was open and seemed to be foaming with some yellowish chalky stuff.

"Nick! What is that?"

He just looked at me. Had he been bitten by a rabid dog? Was he vomiting? Suddenly I knew. Of course. It was his medications. His entire mouth was full of chewed up pills. I stuck my finger in and tried to scoop the crumbles out as I grabbed my phone with the other hand and called Craig.

"I'm at Nick's. He's taken a whole bunch of his medication!" I was whispering for some reason.

"What? I can't understand what you're saying."

"It's Nick. I think he took an overdose. What do I do?"

"We have to get him to the hospital, Miriam!"

Wow. All that NAMI training, and then, because I didn't want to make a scene and get Nick evicted, I decided to drive him to our house and have the paramedics meet us there. This involved little me wrangling a two-hundred-pound, semiconscious man downstairs and into the car. Craig's job was to call 911 and pretend that Nick was there already.

There were two ambulances and a fire truck in front of our house. I was stuck on the corner at the long red light, but even from there I could tell the paramedics were not happy. When I finally got up there, Craig was trying to explain the logic behind summoning them to a place without a patient. A bunch of neighbors watched from their porches.

"Here he is, here he is," I panted. "There, in the car. His mouth is full of pills."

Two of the paramedics jogged to the car.

"Please help him," I said, my voice quavering now. I'd just realized all the time I'd wasted. I had been worried about him being evicted. Now he could die because of that faulty priority. What was wrong with me?

They moved him to the ambulance and took off, sirens blaring, telling me it was serious. Craig and I drove our car. When we got to the hospital, the ambulance was already pulling away. I jumped out and ran up to the guard.

"Where's my son? Is he okay?" I held on to the door handle to steady myself.

"Ma'am, you'll have to go on in to the emergency room. They can get you up to speed." He said this calmly and gently. I was positive that meant Nick was dead.

We rushed into the waiting room and up to the desk.

"Hi, my son, Nick, his name is Nicholas O'Rourke, was just brought in by that ambulance. Where is he? How can we find him?" Craig and I just stood there, planted like trees.

Ten minutes later, we were called to Nick's room. Although they always make the colors cheery in the hospital, a veil of heartache dulls everything, a sorrowful pall you can't escape. The air had the fragrance of flowers, with a knife's sharp edge of rubbing alcohol.

I took a breath tentatively, blinking my eyes. His head was turned to the side, noble profile etched into the pillow, skin the color of earth. He lay in a bed with blue sheets and had a large tube running from some slurping machine down his throat. It was about two inches in diameter and filled with black stuff. There were IV needles stuck in his arms and a cord attached to the tip of his index finger.

The doctor walked in. "Your son has taken a large amount of medication. He is in very serious condition. His blood pressure is dangerously low, and his heartbeat is irregular. We've pumped his stomach, and what you see now is a charcoal solution we are circulating to draw out any residual toxins. He is very lucky that you got him here when you did. A few more minutes, and we would have had to put him on a ventilator." My hand floated up to my mouth as I realized a ventilator would mean he was on life support.

"What happens now?" Craig asked, slowly sitting in a chair. I was bouncing around inside my skin, like a jack-in-the-box as the handle turns, clicking tighter and tighter.

"We wait. Hopefully the charcoal will absorb the rest of the chemicals and he will regain consciousness. It would be very helpful to know what he took, and how much."

Everyone in the room looked at me.

"I don't know," I'm reasonably sure I bellowed. "He takes Zyprexa, and another one, a yellow one. Oh, and I also think he has Aleve at home." *Why hadn't I been keeping better track of all this?*

"Would it be possible to find out?" the doctor asked.

"I'll go. You stay here, Craig. I know where to look." I turned toward the door, looked over my shoulder at my unconscious son, and ran out of the hospital.

Alone in the car, I started to cry. Then I started hyperventilating and had to pull over. I called Brooke and told her what was going on.

"I'm afraid to go in there alone," I said.

"Just take slow breaths and drive over. I'll meet you."

She was standing in front when I pulled up.

"Oh, Mimi, I'm so sorry." She took my arm. I couldn't stop crying.

Although I checked on him daily, he usually met me outside. I hadn't been inside the apartment for months. Huge spiderwebs draped like hammocks from the ceiling. The venetian blinds had a half-inch of dust on every slat. The kitchen counter surface was not even visible; piles and piles of dishes and take-out containers obscured even the sink. Nick had covered the windows with large sheets of black velvet fabric remnants, open only around a whirring fan on the sill. The screen and blades of the once-white fan were black with dirt. On Nick's night table was a mountain of ancient cigarette butts. Burn marks from ashes stippled the carpet. There was trash everywhere. I stopped crying.

We scurried around looking for any kind of pill bottle we could find. There were three empty prescription ones, another one with a few Aleve still in it, and a half-full bottle of the yellow ones. I stuffed them all into my purse.

"Do you want me to follow you to the hospital?" Brooke asked.

"No, Craig's there. I'll call you as soon as I know anything."

She hugged me, I thanked her, and we each drove off. *Thank God for my friends*, I thought. Why did I wait so long to let people help me?

Craig and I sorted through the bottles, did reverse calculations from the bottle quantities on the labels, and tried to figure out what he'd taken. We were helped by James, a strapping young nurse who had recently moved here from the hale and wholesome Midwest.

"People are just more tolerant out here, if you know what I mean," he said. I managed a weak smile and then started crying again.

"Is he going to die?"

"Oh, no, dear, I don't think so," James said. "I'm sure the charcoal will do its job and he'll wake up soon."

Craig and I sat on either side of the bed and looked at our boy. I reached over and smoothed his hair away from the charcoal tube. His cheek was stubbled like a man, but his hair was silken, babylike.

I took out my little flip phone. It had a built-in camera, but I had never used that feature. I was gripped by the thought that if Nick died, I would have no current photograph of him. I hadn't gotten a picture since the ill-conceived portrait at College Hospital. He was still growing. He'd changed a lot since then. I figured the controls out and took several shots. Later, I printed them, and after several years had passed, I started some paintings. The project began well enough, but the process took a turn to a place I wasn't ready to go, I suppose. I realized I couldn't do it. I rolled gesso over them and painted something else. Only I know what is under the new paintings, buried, lost.

"Do you think we should get the girls? I mean, what if . . . like this is the last chance . . ." I couldn't say the words. Lucy was sixteen, Rose almost thirteen.

"No. I don't know," Craig said. "They're still in school. Let's just wait."

The afternoon dragged on. I called Scarlett and, in a hushed monotone, told her what was going on. We were in some sort of fugue state choreographed to the choppy whirrs and clicks of the machinery. James stayed with us. He chattered on to get us through the time. Then, with no fanfare at all, Nick opened his eyes.

"Well, there you are!" James said.

The doctor returned. Nick wasn't going to die, but he was still in serious condition. They would move him to the ICU later that night and then, if all was well, into a room tomorrow. He would be on an involuntary hold, since this did appear to be a suicide attempt. He wouldn't be able to talk until he was extubated. The doctor suggested that we go get some rest.

I scribbled an excessive amount of contact information on James's clipboard as I fumbled with keys, purse, phone. Craig took my elbow and nudged me toward the door. Suddenly a ballerina, I did a slight pirouette back toward the bed to capture the image of my boy, head tilted poetically, flaccid arms strapped at his sides. Asleep, he almost appeared to be lying in state. It was horrible.

We had to go tell the girls. They were older now. It was pointless to try to hide things. When they got into the car, we told them that something had happened with Nick. Then we told them the truth.

Rose was silent. Lucy burst into tears. "Mom, remember Papa," she whimpered.

"No, Lucy. He is not going to die. What happened with Papa, that is not going to happen," I said. Lucy sat forward, her tapered fingers gripping the headrest. Rose slumped in the back seat, fiddling with the strap on her backpack. Craig pulled the car to the curb and stopped. I climbed over into the back seat.

Craig's father had been in the hospital for a broken hip, nothing life-threatening. One evening I went to see him during visiting hours, asking Lucy casually if she wanted to come along. She declined, said she figured she'd see him on the weekend, and sent her love. The next morning, with no warning, we were notified that he had died. The girls were devastated. Lucy was still dealing with that guilty memory now, and I could see the fear in her eyes.

When we returned, Nick was sitting up in the bed. His color was back to normal.

"Hi, guys," he said. A big smile spread gloriously across his handsome face.

Good old James was right there by his side.

"This is James," Nick said, his voice rough from the tube. "He's really funny."

"Hey, girls. Nice to meet you." James smiled.

"What's wrong with your voice?" Lucy stepped past us to the bed, taking Rose's forearm in her left hand, threading her through as well.

"Oh, I'm okay," Nick said. "Don't worry."

Lucy threw herself onto his chest, arms holding the sides of the bed, like a cross. Rose reached out a hand and softly touched one of his fingers.

We all stood around making small talk. There were a million questions to address, but not in front of the girls. Nobody said the word *suicide*. We acted like some unnamed mishap had caused the current situation. Finally, James offered to take them to the vending machines.

"Nick, do you know what happened?" Craig asked. "Do you know why you're here?"

"I'm not sure," he said calmly.

"You took all of your medication!" I said, a little less calmly. "I found you at your apartment, and you were out of it. You answered the door, foaming at the mouth! What did you do?"

He just stared at us and shook his head from side to side. He does that when he wants to check out of a challenging situation.

"Were you trying to kill yourself, Bub?" Craig asked.

At this he seemed to wake up a bit. He explained that it was all a *misunderstanding*. He was definite about not being suicidal. He got "mixed up," he said. He said he thought he might have accidentally taken his meds more than once. We challenged him, and the story kept changing. He was being cagey. Finally, we got it out of him.

"I was doing so well on my medication, I just thought that if I took it all, it might just make me better permanently. You know, like I was before." His eyes were familiar suddenly. Craig turned away with his elbow in one hand, the other covering his face because he was biting his lip, eyes squinched shut, trembling.

We explained more to Lucy and Rose on the way home. Rose silently took it all in, and Lucy howled, "I know this is going to be like Papa! He seems fine, and then he's going to die!"

"He is out of the woods now," Craig said firmly.

"What if he does it again?" She wept.

We attempted to calm her fears, make promises that were true. But we were just winging it. We had the same fears.

The next morning Craig and I returned to find Nick out of intensive care. He had a nurse designated specially to watch over him. There was no guard at the door this time, but he was never left alone. He was in fine spirits, laughing and talking with his nurse. Nick had a pad of paper and was writing furiously.

"Are you kidding?" he asked. "You've never seen *Breathless* by Goddard? That's going on the list!"

She giggled and patted his hand.

"How about *Children of Paradise*?" She shook her head no. Nick scribbled away. I walked over and looked at the pad. He was writing a list:

The Maltese Falcon
Psycho
A Streetcar Named Desire
Midnight Cowboy
Apocalypse Now
The Deer Hunter
Taxi Driver
Raging Bull
Breathless
Children of Paradise

"What is this?" I asked.

"You can't believe it, Ma. Amy has never seen any of these classic films. We started talking about movies, and she's never seen anything. Only stupid ones. So I'm making her a list." He turned and looked at her. "Now you have to promise me you'll rent these. I mean it."

She nodded her head vigorously and continued patting. I sat down just as Craig walked in.

"What's going on?" he asked.

"Don't ask," I said. "Let's just try and get some information here." I pushed the button. Nick and Amy exchanged feigned scared faces and then started laughing.

"What?" I said.

"Oh, now you did it, Mom. You called the mean nurse. She doesn't like us."

"Why would you say that?"

They both looked at the floor, and Nick said, "We got in trouble."

I didn't want to know what that was about and was happy when the mean nurse made a preemptive arrival. She told us what had transpired overnight. Nick was physically out of the woods now. The psychiatrist would decide if the seventy-two-hour hold would be extended.

She also informed us that Nick had been pulling the IVs out of his arm. I started to lecture him about the destructiveness of that, and Craig talked about the dangers of overdosing. We tried, over and over, to make him see the realities. As she tried to replace the needle in his arm, the nurse told him he should listen to his parents. He smiled.

"This has to change, Nick," I said firmly. The nurse was tap, tap, tapping for a vein—a way in. *Join the club*, I thought.

There was blood on the sheets. Syringe after syringe piled up on the bed as she kept trying. The nurse was getting frustrated. I was horrified. Amy stood by, Nick's stalwart companion. Nick asked Craig if he could go get him some candy from the gas station down the street.

"No," Craig snapped. "Are you kidding?"

Finally, the IV was back in place. The nurse stormed out, leaving poor Amy to clean up.

I lost it. "Candy? CANDY? No candy. No rewards, no treats. You don't get good stuff for scaring the shit out of your dad and me. No treats for that, buddy boy." I was yelling.

Nick turned to Amy, who was collecting the broken syringes, and said, "Excuse me, but could I get a couple of those to take home with me?"

"What? What would you need them for?" I rolled my eyes to God.

"Oh," Nick said, "maybe I want to remove the ketchup from some ketchup pouches and replace it with mayonnaise." Amy chuckled. Nick smiled. Craig walked out of the room. I mean, it was funny, the thing about the ketchup. He was messing with us. I got it. Was there any way to reach into that joke and find my son?

When the psychiatrist arrived that afternoon, I was ready. I had all my NAMI instructions chambered.

"I see by his chart that your son has been diagnosed with bipolar, possible schizophrenia, but he appears stable right now. He denies that it was a suicide attempt. I suggest from here on in, you keep the medication and dispense it to him."

I cannot believe that I hadn't already been doing that.

"He's lying," I said. "It was definitely a suicide attempt. He told me last night. He's tried before. You can see the scar under his tattoo. He told me he is going to try again."

Lies? Yes. But the guidelines for having a person hospitalized against their will are extremely stringent, and I wasn't going to make a mistake. The patient must meet one of three criteria:

1. They must be an imminent danger to themselves.
2. They must be an imminent threat to the safety of others.
3. They must be unable to care for themselves.

The first two are very clear. Number three is much narrower than it may seem. By "unable to care for themselves," the guidelines are not referring to the lack of a nice haircut or matching socks. It means they literally cannot feed themselves or provide for their essential needs because they are that crazy. It's a hard one to meet, which is why we usually go with danger to themselves or others. Dr. Warner frowned at me. He knew what I was doing. The next day they sent Nick back to College Hospital. His stay was extended until Monday, when there would be a hearing to determine if he could leave. I was ecstatic. Any time in a psychiatric facility offered hope and, selfishly, some modest respite from immediate crisis preparedness for me.

The task at hand was to gird my loins and go back to Nick's apartment; it was cleaning time. Armed with every supply imaginable, I scrubbed, vacuumed, and pulled spiderwebs from the walls. The bathroom was revolting, like the worst bus terminal. There were legions of cockroaches in the sink. I smashed them with my bare hands. I filled bag after bag with trash. The crazy, surprising thing was—I loved it. *I loved it.* This I could do. I couldn't fix his brain. I couldn't slay his demons. I couldn't trade places with him. But I could clean that goddamned apartment.

Job done, I closed the door behind me and walked out into the afternoon sun. As I thought about Nick's expression when he told us why he'd taken the pills, a scrawny cat skittered across the street. The air smelled faintly of smoke.

I could still smell the smoke as I pulled into my driveway. I could see it in the sky above the studio, maybe a fire in the hills. Craig was in his shop, the early afternoon sun articulating the teeth of the table saw, the curve of his neck, his hands. The shop was all open space and glass. No posts held the ceiling up. He had designed it that way, constructing massive trusses to distribute the roof's weight. I remember him lovingly sanding the numerous gussets that hold it together, as though each were an art piece.

"Wow, that's a lot of plaques."

"They're called gussets," he'd said, smiling to himself.

"Well, why are you hand sanding them? Why are you even sanding them at all? They're never going to be touched way up there. No one will know . . ."

"I will know," he'd said, his smile lingering.

Craig walked down the driveway with Buster to meet me. "Is there a fire?"

"Must be," I said.

"So how did it go?"

"You don't want to know. It's clean now. That's what matters."

"What are we going to do?"

"He's gone, Craig. He's somewhere else . . ."

I could see the smoke everywhere now, interrupting the sun's light, making the day a shade darker. We looked at each other. I had such a thickness in my throat there was no way to talk. We put our arms around each other, my face reached his flannel shirt just above the solar plexus, and I pushed it in there. I wanted to go inside.

Both of us sobbed, shedding pretense, letting misery loose. Buster tiptoed around us, whining and sniffing the air.

We entered another time of relative calm. I drove to Nick's every day to give him his meds, a pack of cigarettes, and ten dollars. I'd call him on my way so he could wait outside—it saved time. It was a strange ritual: me pulling up in my truck, loaded with ladders and paint, him sauntering over to take his pills.

It was different every day. Sometimes he was cheery and talkative.

"Hey, Ma, how's it going?" He'd peer in the window.

Other days he was completely out of it, disheveled hair and expression, mumbling. The worst was when he'd appear, eyes flat and cold, wordlessly take his provisions, and then turn away. Sometimes he'd jerk his hand just as I was depositing the pills so one would fall to the ground.

"I can't take that one now. Give me another."

"Nick, I have only a certain amount of these. You have to stop doing this. Why can't you just cup your hand like a normal person?" I actually said that: *like a normal person*. Oh yes.

After he'd go inside, I'd crawl under the truck, retrieve the pill, and put it back in the bottle.

After a month he seemed better. He'd put the pills in his mouth and then hold out his hand for the money. "Swallow them, Nick," I'd order. "Open your mouth and let me see, now lift up your tongue." Once I knew the medicine was in his stomach, I could go on with my day.

HE CAME IN WITH IT

Lucy was sprawled on the daybed in my workroom looking at college applications. I was at my table, making color samples for a mural I was designing.

"Can I get on the computer?" Rose appeared at the door wearing the hat from the tree costume I'd made her for Halloween, green felt leaves of varying shades framing her oblong face, heavy-lidded eyes calling up the mystery of the forest.

"Yeah, sure," I said.

"Rose, do you want to drive up to Santa Barbara with me and check out the school this weekend?" Lucy asked.

"No, because you are not going to college. You can't leave me here alone with this crazy woman."

"Oh, thanks," I said, flicking some water her way from my brush.

"You won't be alone. Dad will be here," Lucy offered.

"Oh, right. He doesn't live here anymore."

"Rose, I wish you wouldn't say that. Your dad lives here. He's working on the house up north for all of us."

Rose rolled her eyes, Lucy cleared her throat, and I busied myself with some white paint as if my life depended on it.

The days went by. The pharmaceuticals were measured and dispensed. I tried to be grateful for all the sunsets and all the colors. I painted fiendishly, desperately, shoving the pain of Nick away from me as paint flew everywhere. Every day was a battle, followed by a couple of glasses of red wine at night.

But the pain lurked. It was like a big old dog outside a closed back door. Sometimes he would look at me with his large, sad eyes. Sometimes he whined. Other days he'd sleep and not bother me at all. Occasionally I had to let him in; I just couldn't stand it. I'd open the door with resignation and say in a long, exaggerated sigh, "All right, tonight you can come in." And every single time it was the same thing. That old dog ripped the place to pieces.

8

BLOODWALLS

Nick had been quiet since the overdose. He would sit on the porch during his visits to the house. As a child, I had loved *To Kill a Mockingbird*, and my favorite character was Boo Radley. How he captured my imagination. The misunderstood misfit whose goodness prevailed. Now, decades later, I had my own Boo Radley.

Nick came to the house for Father's Day dinner and never said a word. That seemed to be all right with everybody. At least he wasn't making noises or saying creepy things. But I wanted to holler, to keep asking him questions until he cracked open and revealed who he had been before he got sick.

"So, Nick," I said loudly, "are you happy right now?" I put down my fork.

He gave me the slow head shake.

"Are you unhappy? Are you sad?"

"No," he said softly.

"Then what is it? If you're not unhappy, then things are fine? You're content?" I demanded, like an aggressive attorney.

"Sure."

Everyone at the table stared at me with varying degrees of open mouths.

"What?" I barked. "You all just act like nothing's wrong. Well, that's not okay with me."

"What does that even mean?" Lucy said.

"It means never give up, baby," I declared.

Lucy and Rose giggled. Mom was losing it.

"Nicknack," I asked, "are you ready to go home?"

He shook his head no and said, "Yes."

In the car, his placid demeanor conjured up Boo once again. I glanced at my side-view mirror and noticed the sky. The day had maybe an hour or so left. A fair, yellow-white sun rested on the June horizon. That sun was so immaculate and so fresh, it bleached the whole sky around to match its strange color. I stared in the mirror at that elegance. I wanted to disappear into it. I didn't dare look away from the mirror to the actual sky.

A couple weeks earlier, Nick hadn't been so serene. I arrived at his place for my weekly cleanliness inspection and found several fist-sized holes in the walls.

"What in the world?" I was confused. "How did this happen? Where did these holes come from?"

Nick looked down.

"I'm serious. Did you do this?" I glared at him, and then he glared right back.

"Let me see your hands, Nick."

Reluctantly he held them out; his knuckles were bruised purple and raw. I felt sick. "You punched the walls?"

"No, no, I didn't do that. It's just sometimes, with my medication, you know. I get anxious and bang into things. It was an accident."

"An accident? Three times?"

"It's just a misunderstanding, Mom."

"A misunderstanding that is going to get you evicted! If you make a problem here, you have nowhere to go. Let me see those hands." After cleaning and wrapping his hands as much as he would allow, I went home. I told him I'd be back shortly. I returned with a bucket of plaster and two six-inch flexible mud knives.

"I've got to fix these, man. Right now," I said. "And you are going to help me." I handed him a knife. I had to prompt him for every move, but we worked side by side.

The holes would reappear periodically, and I'd lug some plaster over. The cause ceased to be a subject of discussion. I just spackled them up and painted over them.

The day after the first repair job, I went over to take him to his appointment at Kaiser. I still wasn't thrilled with the care he was receiving, but there were no other options. He was bad that week, angry with me after the wall thing. We drove up a street I had driven him many times as a baby, a boy, a teenager. Only this time, the person in my car was a scary, scary stranger.

He began to rant. He yelled, and he banged his wrists together and made strange guttural noises. He kicked his leg over and over, slammed his head against the seat. He spoke gibberish.

He began to yell the same word over and over: "*Hajima. Hajima. Hajima.*" Louder and louder he screamed and banged and slammed.

I drove as if frozen, unable to process what was happening.

Hajima was a word I remembered. It's a Korean word the kids used to say when they were younger. I didn't know what it meant or why he was saying it; was he trying to reach into his childhood?

I sat in the driver's seat beside my son, his eyes bugging out, unearthly sounds filling the car. Was he going to hit me? Grab the steering wheel?

Suddenly, he jumped out of the car and into traffic, then ran screaming down the street. Calf turning to ankle, rooted in foot, he flew. I watched him until he moved out of the street onto the sidewalk. *Where he was safe.*

I have since learned what *hajima* means: stop it.

I could see his anguish, railing at the universe that had done this unspeakable thing to him. I could see the shadow of the boy within the contour of the man he had become. Stunned into temporary numbness, I drove away.

All around the city, there are buildings where someone decided that a window should be closed up. A worker comes and uses stucco to fill it in. It always looks good at first. But time passes, and gradually the thing happens that always happens—the shape of what had been there reappears. It always bleeds through. There is only one way to truly get rid of it: tear off the entire wall. You have to stucco the whole damn thing, from scratch coat to finish coat, in order to make the phantom window go away. Why is that? Why is it so hard to just patch something up?

My stupefaction wore off, like Novocain after the dentist, and by the time I reached Kaiser I was pretty hysterical. I made a scene, begged the receptionist to help me. They took me into one of those overly bright and lively rooms, where I was counseled by a social worker. He was very understanding but offered me nothing. As soon as was possible, they ushered me out.

I never found out where Nick ran off to. I called him later at home, and he acted like nothing had happened, then hung up on me. Click. I was used to it, but each time Nick left the line it had a weird, special kind of fade out, like he'd exited into another world. I swear sometimes I could hear vague electrical noises, whistles, like ghosts.

I lived in Israel for several years as a teenager. My mother, devastated by her divorce, immigrated there with my brother and me. I returned to the states when I came of age, yearning for a life I mistakenly thought I could reclaim.

There is a wind that blows in Israel called the *hamsin*. It's hot and heavy and makes everybody uncomfortable. Yellow sand would hit the air and turn a blue sky suddenly white. I remember when those winds would blow. They would come as though burst from a dam— angry and hot—and then vanish. In California, we have the Santa Ana winds. They're similar but without the sand. Usually they visit us in the fall. It was one of those days. My friend Carolyn was having a barbecue.

We sat in her garden, and I surveyed the group around me. Carolyn had two sons about Nick's age, so the place was alive with youthful exuberance. It was difficult not to veer into comparisons in those days. There they were, the healthy ones, full of future. It took serious effort to avoid wallowing. But I did it. Lucy and Rose lit up my day, and I was surrounded with friends. I had to allow myself to enjoy what was good. We left after a few hours, well-fed and happy.

I started to have a bad feeling. I tried to shake it off. It hung on. I called Nick, and there was no answer. Not unusual—he often slept during the day or just checked out for long periods of time. But my anxiety increased, and I called again. No answer. When I got home, I called for what felt like a thousand times before deciding I had to go over there. This happened a lot. I'd run over because I had some terrible premonition, and he'd open the door, all sleepy and disheveled. I'd say, "Oh, Nick. Just wanted to say hi. See you later," and then I'd drive home feeling foolish but knowing it was like the tide, this pull. There was no fighting it.

I was already admonishing myself as I knocked on his door. There was a thump of a noise and then nothing. By now it was almost dark out. I knocked again. After some shuffling, he opened the door. He stood there, leaning against the wall, in his boxer shorts. It was shadowy, and against the windows he was a silhouette.

"Nick! What the hell? Why don't you ever answer your phone?"

"Huh? Uh, I don't know. I was resting," he mumbled.

"Are you all right? You seem kind of out of it." I still had a funny feeling. "I can't even see you. Turn on the light."

I slid my arm in next to him and pushed the switch up.

He was completely covered in blood. As the synapses of my brain scrambled to take this in, I realized the walls were also smeared red.

"Oh my God, Nick, what happened?"

He staggered a little and said nothing.

I didn't know where to begin. *Where was the blood coming from? Had he hurt himself? Had someone else attacked him? Oh God, was this someone else's blood?*

"Come over here and sit on the bed." I got calm. I surveyed his body and could find no origin for the blood. Is it possible to feel relief and abject terror at the same time? If this blood was not flowing from Nick, what the hell had happened?

I dialed 911, then sat down on the bed next to my gory boy and took in the scene around me. Waiting on a sagging mattress for rescue, he leaned his shoulder slightly against me, and I held his weight. We sat there like some kind of macabre pietà. Within minutes, the paramedics arrived. They examined him and found a large crack on the back of his head.

"The scalp bleeds very profusely, ma'am. It may not be as bad as it seems," Hero-Fireman-Whom-I-Will-Love-Forever said.

"Sir, please turn this way so we can bandage your head before we take you to the hospital," Gentle-Paramedic-Whom-I-Would-Die-For said.

I marvel at this world in which we live. We walk a planet where it is possible to pick up a small electronic device, press some buttons, and tall, strong men and women come to help. They don't look around the room and see the cockroaches and grime and leave in disgust. They called me "ma'am." They called him "sir." Their cordial and uncomplaining civility was a deeply felt blessing. The property might have been worthy of being condemned, but they did not condemn its inhabitants.

Onto the gurney and into the ambulance. This was the second time I watched him loaded into that red-and-white truck.

"What do I do?" I asked. "Do I go in the ambulance with you?"

"No, ma'am. It's better if you can follow in your car so you will have means of transportation from the hospital."

Oh, I knew that. I called the girls and told them I was taking Nick out for a sandwich.

Outside, the winds still blew, and then, for a moment, they stopped. The land felt frozen. The stillness was so complete that the sky and the earth and all of the trees, even the rocks, rested in halcyon splendor. The heat, which remained in the air, somehow lost its warmth. I looked at my bloody hands as the ambulance pulled away. I stood with my face to the heavens and waited. The wind resumed, and I went to the hospital.

Once there, he got a raft of stitches. He was going to be fine, physically; I brought them up to speed on all the psychiatric stuff. They asked him if it had been a suicide attempt. He said no, he didn't know how it had happened. I had a suspicion he'd slammed his head against the wall. I told them it was definitely a suicide attempt, and not the first, and insisted they bring the psychiatrist. Which they did. Relief. I had seventy-two hours to regroup.

After calling Craig from the car, I went home. I didn't tell Lucy and Rose about this one. It was too appalling. They didn't need those images in their heads. I went upstairs and poured myself a glass of wine, which I now kept in the sewing cabinet in my work-room. Looking at the mail, I saw another jury summons for Nicholas O'Rourke. For crying out loud, was this a joke?

The next day, I woke with a certainty like none I'd had before. All this was my fault. Not because of anything I did while I was preg-nant. Not from the fall on his head at my brother's. *It was because I had been prideful.* Nick was so handsome, so talented, so smart. I had taken pleasure in comparing him to other kids, and God had given him this illness to punish me. It was my fault.

I wandered through that day in a state of self-loathing. I wanted to die. I called Theresa, the friend to whom I could reveal ugly secrets. I poured out the whole story, my long-overdue epiphany, and then just sobbed.

"Oh, darling, please stop. This just isn't so," she cooed to me over the phone. "I know how you feel. I know what you're saying, but it's just your mind playing tricks on you. It's all so gruesome you can't process it. Please believe me, this is not your fault."

Whoever's fault all this was, I sure as hell knew who was going to have to clean it up.

I really do believe that there is nothing so terrible in this world that it cannot be handled with a pair of Playtex Living Gloves. I didn't attempt anything in Nick's apartment without them anymore. I was dreading seeing the place in the daylight, but I wanted to get it over with.

It looked like a murder scene. There was blood all over: splattered on the walls, on his bed, on the floor—everywhere. This was the same blood that had flooded the delivery room table the day he was born, his and mine, mixed. I began. I had a bucket, hot water, ammonia, scrubbing brushes. I didn't cry this time. Something about the addition of blood to the mix put it in another category. Tears seemed meager.

As I arched to the long strokes it required to scrub walls, cleansing, salty sweat ran down my face. I moved around on my hands and knees, furiously scouring the floor with my brush. Stopping for a second to wipe sweat, I realized again, *I like this. I am doing something. When I finish, the blood will be gone. At this, I am at last effective.*

I called the county courthouse to discuss the jury summons issue. I mean, three summonses in two years? Each time I made up some excuse, but clearly this wasn't going to end. I sat on hold for forty-five minutes and finally got an actual person—one Ms. Morgan. I explained the situation in detail so she would understand that Nick would never be a juror.

"Oh, honey, you don't need to speak with me. You need to call the Office of Permanent Excuses!"

"The *what?*" I was sure I hadn't heard correctly.

"It's the way to get him off the juror list for good," Ms. Morgan said, and with that, the magic phone number was mine.

Wait, what? Who knew? The Office of Permanent Excuses. That could be useful to a person in so many ways. I let myself ponder my many transgressions over the years, all the things of which I am ashamed. Perhaps this enchanted office could be of some help to me as well? I sure would like to be excused from oh so many of my duties. How much time did they have for my petitions?

I dialed the number. A woman—not a recording—answered. "Office of Permanent Excuses, how may I help you?"

Oh, the list I had already made in my head of my endless fuckups. "Yes, hello. My name is Miriam Feldman, and my son, Nick, is mentally ill. He has gotten three jury summonses in the past two years, and he really isn't ever going to be able to be on a—"

She cut me off right there. "Well, you need a 1644 form, which will have to be signed by his doctor, and that will take him out of the rotation. Would you like me to mail it to you?"

"Yes, that would be great," I said, and gave her the address.

"Is there anything else I can help you with?" she asked.

"Um, yeah . . . do you deal with . . . other things as well?" I couldn't help myself.

"I'm not sure I understand what you mean, ma'am." She was a little curt, I have to say.

"Oh, nothing, never mind. Thank you so much for your time," I said, and hung up, smiling, always my own best audience.

Kaiser had decided to cut all Medi-Cal patients from psychiatric care, so I had to find help elsewhere. I went to the County Department of Mental Health. It was located across from MacArthur Park, where I used to go see the baby ducks when I was a kid. Now it was the outdoor campground of junkies and criminals. Appointments? Oh, no. You just go there and wait. The waiting room was a tableau of all that is good and evil in the universe.

Completely insane people ran around freely, unrestrained. Determined family members sat and waited patiently. Little babies and children wandered about unsupervised. There were many vacant-eyed old people sitting, looking lost. It *really* smelled in there—body odor, rancid sweat, food, urine, and old cigarettes. In one corner of the large room sat a tall, very thin man of about fifty. He was wearing filthy chinos and a once-white shirt. At his feet lay an old-fashioned bedroll. To the left, on the floor, sat a cardboard box with a large, half-eaten sheet cake in it.

The people who worked there ran the gamut. There were the fervent beginners, still certain they would make a difference. The diligent professionals, some guardedly optimistic, others already disillusioned. Ah, and the journeymen, the ones who had been at it forever, with empty eyes and presumably defeated hearts. Nick was assigned a counselor, Josh.

Josh was a novice and about Nick's age. I felt ridiculous sitting across the desk from him, like I should reach over and fix his collar or something. As Nick's counselor, he'd do home visits (*have fun, Josh*) and take him out for exercise and activities.

The Josh/Nick experiment worked for a while. Josh got him out of his apartment and took a little of the pressure off me for social engagement. But at County they didn't monitor medication, which was important. Then I remembered young Dr. Jeremy Hamill, who had first diagnosed him. After hours of Google searching, I located him. He wasn't seeing patients anymore; he was working on clinical trials. If we could convince Nick to participate in one, he could oversee it and perhaps get Nick on some new miracle drug that would cure him! He didn't actually say the miracle drug part, but that's what I heard. He might also end up getting the placebo, but Dr. Hamill had no control over that. It was risky, because then he'd be off all meds. We were scared of what might happen.

Craig and I were standing in the kitchen one day, and he gently admonished me not to leave sharp knives out on the counter when Nick was around. I wanted to be mad at him, but he was right.

I thought of a conversation I'd recently had with a friend.

"Oh, I don't worry about violence. Nick would never hurt a fly." Who was I kidding? Nick was crazy. I was scared to death. All the time. Awake in the middle of the night, I'd recall the sticky, sweet blood on his walls and my terror about the source. I worried about the burn marks on the carpet and accidental fires and missed pills. How the hell were the girls ever going to get over this? And had he hurt anyone? Would he kill himself? And who is going to take care of him when I'm dead? And would the girls develop schizophrenia? And what the fuck was that lump behind my knee?

I fumbled along with Nick. One day he came out to the car with a black eye, no explanation. He'd show up with odd injuries and just blankly shake his head if I pressed him on it. For a week, he kept his hoodie up, so I didn't see he'd shaved his head. Whenever I saw the cracked, red knuckles, I knew it was plaster time. Once he accidentally dropped *all* of his Zyprexa in the street and then refused to take any of them. I frantically tried cleaning them off, but he wouldn't budge. He had a purple-and-yellow smudge of a bruise on his cheekbone, a burnt sienna swirl of nicotine staining the palm he held up as he said, "No."

I drove up to Rite Aid to throw myself at the mercy of the pharmacist. It was common knowledge by then in the neighborhood that there was "something wrong with Nick." Our good friends knew everything, but most people really didn't want to know.

It was my turn at the counter. "Hi. Listen, I have kind of a problem here. You know my son, Nick, I get his medications here? Well, they spilled on the ground, and now he won't take them, and he can't go a day without them. It screws everything up. It's after hours now, and I can't reach his doctor."

"Oh, that's okay, we can give you a carry-over prescription for the weekend," he said. "Just wait over there, and we'll call you over when they're ready."

A carry-over prescription?

I felt such a rush of relief I was lightheaded. I turned and saw my friend Robin in the next aisle. "Hi," she said. "Long time no see!"

Of course, I started bawling. Don't ever be nice to me, or I will start bawling. She put her arms around me, and we stood in the middle of Rite Aid, a spectacle.

The rock-lined hills of central California seemed endless on the ride up to UC Santa Cruz, where Lucy had decided to go for college. I wanted it to be like the commercials—colorful storage containers filled with new school supplies, excited kid, teary parents. I counted on Lucy to provide us with a taste of the life portrayed on TV, a life now far out of my reach.

After a choreographed weekend, we stood in front of the dorms saying goodbye. When it was Rose's turn, she clung to Lucy for a long time. Lucy buried her face in Rose's hair and whispered quietly. Rose peeled herself away, glared and Craig and me, and walked sadly toward the parking lot.

"She is taking this hard," Craig said.

"I am going to make it up to her." I watched her small frame disappear behind a tall redwood. "Now I am going to give her the attention she deserves. I'm going to turn this thing around."

I had it all figured out. I realized she must have felt invisible with the drama going on around her, that she hadn't gotten the mother the other kids had: Ridgewood Place Mom, confident, strong, attentive. She's gotten Broken Mom, and I intended to fix that. There was only one problem: it was becoming increasingly apparent that she already hated me and had for a while.

When I wasn't driving the sullen, noncommunicative Rose around to every kind of lesson or activity I could think of to make her happy, I was trying to find Nick a new doctor. He didn't want to meet with Josh anymore. He was getting skittish about taking his meds, so when he said, "You know, Ma, it's the weekend, and I would really like to relax and have a beer. It would calm me down and make it easier for me to stay on my meds." I heard the threat. Maybe he *was* crazy like a fox.

I hit the internet to see how beer would interact with his current cocktail of pills. It didn't seem harmful in moderation, so the Friday night beer ritual was born. Until then, we were firm in the agreement: a roof over his head, a pack of cigarettes, and ten dollars was his payment for staying on the drugs. When I added beer, I opened the portal for bargaining.

I agreed to buy Nick two bottles of beer on Fridays, and he decided on Mickey's Big Mouth because they were, well, big. I had to make a special stop at the 7-Eleven, and that was a pain. What with ferrying Rose to art workshops, dates with friends, and some weird blues guitar teacher she'd found on the other side of town, I didn't have much spare time. One evening when I was at Safeway picking up groceries, I noticed they carried Mickey's. *Ah ha*, I thought, *if I stock up, then I won't have to do the 7-Eleven run on Fridays!*

I proceeded to fill my cart with an obscene number of beer bottles. Shocking because of the amount, but also because Mickey's is not exactly the Dom Pérignon of beer. It's pretty much the beverage of choice for bums and runaway kids. As I pushed my now-very-heavy cart toward the checkout, the wheels slowly lumbering under the weight of all that glass and fluid, I came face-to-face with Martin and Jane, my friend Laura's kids.

"Uh, hi, Mrs. O'Rourke," Jane said, both of them trying not to stare at my cart.

"Hi, kids. How are you?" I tried to sound natural.

We all stood there, looking everywhere but at the cart, until finally I put us out of our misery. "Well, gotta go. Say hello to your mother!"

Of course, Laura called me later that night. "Hi, honey, how's it going?"

"The beer, right?" I figured, Why waste time?

I told her what the deal was, and she told me how appalled her kids had been. We laughed for a bit and then got down to the serious things. Even Laura, who worked in the mental health field, couldn't offer up much.

Craig and I went around and around the clinical trial idea. We decided it was too much of a risk. I called Dr. Hamill, and he understood. We were saying goodbye when he stopped.

"Wait, I have an idea," he said. "I have a friend, a guy I did my residency with, who is a cutting-edge psychopharmacologist. He has a practice in Beverly Hills, but he volunteers at the Inglewood Mental Health Center. Is Nick on Medi-Cal?"

I said that he was.

"Then he could see him through the clinic, and it would be covered! Believe me, Mimi, you'll never find anyone better than Rod Amiri. Let me just call him," he said. "We'll cut through the red tape."

And with those words, the horrible bus to Crazytown we'd been on took a turn toward the light.

"Dr. Hamill," Craig said. "I always liked the cut of that man's jib."

9

PURE HEART

Nick and I drove to the worst part of Los Angeles.

"I don't get it, Nick," I said. "I don't see anything. Do you?" He didn't answer.

I had promised I'd take him to lunch if he would come with me to see Dr. Amiri. His behavior had become more erratic lately. One day he'd be fine, and the next it'd be the eyes, lined in red. I looked around and saw a large vacant lot with a double-wide trailer in it. Some cars were parked around. Inglewood Mental Health was printed on a piece of paper taped to the door.

"Well, I guess this is it," I said. "Let's go in and meet Dr. Amiri."

Inside the trailer was a paltry attempt at a medical center, to be sure, but after the County office, anything was acceptable. The heavily made-up girl at the folding table took our information and gave me a pile of forms to fill out. I had arrived prepared, bringing a twelve-page history of Nick's illness, including all hospitalizations, medications, and a general summary of the trajectory of his sickness. I had it neatly organized in a plastic folder. No one ever actually read it, but I always brought it.

"You can go in now," the receptionist said, nodding to the other side of the trailer. In?

A good-looking young man in shirtsleeves sat behind a beat-up desk.

"Hello," he said as he stood, holding out his hand. "I'm Dr. Amiri."

I shook his hand, Nick nodded, and we sat.

"It's so nice to meet you," I said. "Dr. Hamill speaks highly of you."

I gave him a brief overview of our situation, and without much hope offered him the folder. Dr. Amiri *was* interested in my tedious chronicle. In fact, he read it right there while we waited.

"May I keep this?"

I couldn't believe my ears. "Of course."

"Nick," he said, "I see that you've been on the Zyprexa for some time now. How is that working for you?"

"Um, I feel a lot of restlessness sometimes, and I have trouble sleeping." Wait. What? He's talking to the doctor about how he feels? What was happening?

"Well, I think we could address some of that by lowering your dosage and adding another medication. Would you be open to that?" he asked Nick.

"Sure," he said.

Dr. Amiri turned to me and said, "I think it is time to address this as schizophrenia. All the criteria are present."

So it had been schizophrenia all along.

It had a name. It was named. The ball had landed at the farthest end of the spectrum.

I remembered standing in the alley behind the restaurant I was painting, warm wind on my skin, getting his first diagnosis of bipolar. I think I knew it was schizophrenia even then.

Nick was looking at his shoe. He didn't seem to hear.

"I think that lithium, which is a mood stabilizer, in combination with an antipsychotic, would work well for Nick. I'd like to give this a try."

"Okay. Whatever you think is best."

"This will be a process of trial and error," he said. "We may have to try several things before we find what's best for him. Also, as time passes, its effectiveness can change. The vital component is to stay on top of it, watch his symptoms, and take the time to understand what he is feeling. We're all going to work together to figure this out. Is that okay with you, Nick?"

"Sure," he said softly.

I wanted to ask him if he had heard the doctor say schizophrenia but was afraid to say the word again.

After lunch, I dropped Nick at his apartment. He usually went into what the family refers to as a *food coma* after he ate and required a nap. I drove quickly to the pharmacy with my crisp new prescription, full of hope.

It took a very long time. I started bringing him his medication in the evenings, along with a plate of whatever I'd made for dinner so he didn't have to come to the house to eat. His behavior was erratic, so it had gotten difficult to have him around.

One night I drove down with a plate of macaroni and cheese covered in cellophane and an apple. He stood scowling on the corner.

"Hi, Nick," I said.

Not saying a word, he took his meds, and I handed him the money and cigarettes. I reached over to hand him the food. "I don't want that," he said angrily.

"Okay, see ya later," I said, setting the plate down on the passenger seat. I didn't argue anymore. Driving home, I looked for a homeless woman I'd noticed. She lived along a wide patch of parkway on my route. She was tall and skinny and had the requisite shopping cart, ripped-up tent, and piles of God knows what. She'd sit with her legs straight out in front of her, reading a book. Sometimes she was pacing up and down, arms thrashing, talking out loud. I'd seen her peeing, giving herself a bath from a bucket, and sleeping all bundled up in grungy blankets.

"Hey. Hello," I called out the window. She started, then looked suspiciously at me. "Are you hungry?" I asked. "I have some dinner here."

She walked slowly to the car, and I held out the plate. "Look, mac and cheese. It's my specialty."

Her face was leathery and her eyes wide-set, hair blonde. She took the plate and said, "Thank you." She walked away and then turned back for a second. "You got any money?"

"Nope," I said truthfully. I never brought my purse when I took Nick his stuff to eliminate the possibility of him asking me for extra money.

It started with his rejects, then before I knew it, I found myself preparing two plates each night.

"What are you doing?" Craig asked.

"It's for Mom's new friend, Deeeeee." Rose smirked. "Mom has a homeless friend now."

"Care to explain?" he asked.

I told him about Dee's encampment. "Oh, I always make too much food anyway. She's so sad, Craig, I felt like such a creep driving right by her with food for Nick. It just doesn't seem fair. He's nuts, she's nuts, but only he gets dinner?"

"You're something else, Feldy," he said, shaking his head in bemusement. "Wait, you know her name?"

"Well, of course I do. I'm not going to just toss food out the window and drive away. She's not an animal in a zoo. We talk."

"They talk," Craig said to Rose, exchanging a knowing look.

Actually, I'd gotten to know quite a bit about Dee. The very first thing she told me, unasked, was that she didn't have schizophrenia.

"Okay," I said. "Neither do I. You've got a nice little setup here."

Dee was from outside Chicago. She'd come out here for the warm weather. She liked to read and believed in bathing daily. Most folks just left her alone, but she liked me, she said. She told me things about her childhood. She'd grown up in a small town and used to be really good at softball. I never did get the story of how she ended up on the streets. She did like to talk about her family. She'd show me what she was reading. There was no continuity to it; she must have just found the books. I'd told her my name a few times, but for some reason she called me Mike.

"See ya later, Dee!"

"Good night, Mike!"

I brought Nick to see Dr. Amiri every three weeks. He adjusted the medication several times, and we started seeing results. It was so exacting, getting it right. Some of the pills had to be cut in half. I learned that there was a special little contraption for doing that, and I bought one.

He took the time to ask Nick a lot of questions about how he was feeling. Privacy laws prohibited doctors from speaking to anyone but the patient about his care without a written release. Some doctors strictly adhere to that, which is fine, but in the case of mental illness it can be very problematic. The doctor's hands are tied, and ours are useless.

At NAMI, they taught us a way around some of this. The law forbids the doctor from disseminating private information, but it does not restrict them from receiving data. The good doctors, the ones who go the extra mile, work with you. They listen. A kind of code develops, like this: "If I ask you this question and you say nothing, I'm going to assume the answer is no."

I got into a groove. I made sure both Nick and Dee had a hot meal every night. Rose directed all her anger in my direction, but I understood. I continued my campaign of earnest and infinite patience and unreserved availability. My campaign of love. Craig came and went; the house in Washington was coming along, and he was now talking about getting some chickens. Business was good, and I was busy. I was working on an elaborate mural in a massive estate up on a hill overlooking the Beverly Hills Hotel. It was an octagonal playroom for a four-year-old girl. I was covering the walls with swinging monkeys and foliage, the ceiling was to have a transition of day on one side to night on the other, complete with sun, stars, and moon.

One morning I was trying to get an early start. My vehicle was set up like a rolling pharmacy/emergency center. All Nick's meds were in a box in the glove compartment. There were water bottles to make sure he swallowed. I had cartons of cigarettes, Band-Aids, Neosporin, and, yes, a pair of Playtex Living Gloves. But it was Friday, and I didn't have any more Mickey's.

Okay, I'll just run by the 7-Eleven on the way, I thought. *There will still be time.*

A long queue went from the register to the back of the store. Who knew so many people were out buying stuff at 6:00 a.m.? After grabbing two enormous green bottles of beer, I took my place in the line. When at last I reached the front and plopped the beers loudly onto the counter, I was met by the disdainful countenance of the cashier. *Oh. 6:00 a.m. Beer. Right.*

"Oh, these aren't for *me*, not at all. I mean who drinks beer at this time of day?" I giggled nervously. Cold stare from him.

"You don't understand. They're for my son!" Well, that certainly didn't make it any better.

"No, you see, my son has schizophrenia, and this is how I get him to take his medicine." I couldn't stop. My shrill, defensive voice filled the store, which had gotten very quiet. I recognized one of my neighbors in line with coffee and a donut. "Sometimes you just gotta do what you gotta do . . . to . . ." Oh, the hell with it. I paid hastily, grabbed the beers, and left.

Sitting in the car with sweat running down my temples, I remembered that Dr. Amiri just changed the lithium to a half dose, and I was supposed to have cut the pills last night. Now what? I tore the car apart looking for something to cut the pills with. Cigarettes flew everywhere. I emptied the contents of the console all over the seat and finally found a nail clipper.

That'll do it! I thought gleefully. I held the pill up in front of my face, squinting to focus, and slid it halfway into the clipper. It turns out that cutting a small pill in half with a nail clipper is harder than you'd think. I went through pill after pill. Some disintegrated, some went flying. I was in a frenzy. In the rearview mirror, I could see that my face was covered with white dust. Nice. At last, I got one to cut. The other part went out the window, but I saved half.

Just at that moment, I looked up and saw two policemen walking past my car. This is what they saw: a middle-aged woman in tattered paint clothes with a nail clipper in her mouth and a big grin. White powder all over her face. The passenger seat was a pile of junk pulled from the console. Cigarette packs were everywhere. On her lap was a bag containing two Mickey's Big Mouths. They paused for a nano-second and then went on their way.

Los Angeles.

Nick mentioned, casually, that the water in his bathroom sink wouldn't turn off.

"Great, how long has that been going on?"

"About a week," he said.

"A week?" I cried. "Why didn't you say something? It must be flooded!"

"There's a little bit of water."

I heaved a sigh loud enough to make sure God heard me, opened the car door, and stared into Nick's hollow eyes. "Let's go see."

The whole bathroom floor was wet. The carpet in the hallway was wet. It stunk like an old public bathhouse in there. I turned off the water at the angle stop, surveyed the squalor, then fought back an urge to punch a few holes in the walls myself.

"For Christ's sake, look at this place," I shouted. "We can't even call the landlord to get a plumber in to fix it. He'll take one look and evict you. At any rate, we better get that carpet dry first."

I started to berate him about the impoverishment of his existence. I knew the unfairness as well as the absurdity of this. I simply had too many needs crashing around inside me. He stood there and quietly reminded me, "Now, don't overreact, Mom." How I loved hearing that in situations to which it was impossible to react *enough*.

"Okay, this is it. I am not going to clean this place myself. I'm calling a cleaning service," I announced defiantly.

"I'm not really sure if I'm comfortable with strangers coming in here, Ma."

"Oh really? You're not comfortable?" I asked. "Well, don't 'over-react,' because it's *going down*. Tomorrow!" I stormed out of his place without even looking at the kitchen.

I googled "cleaning services Los Angeles." Let's see, Merry Maids. Maid This. Clean Sweep. Mission Maids. That's it, that sounded good. Maids on a mission. It felt right. I set it up for the next morning. The place would get clean, and I wouldn't have to lift a finger. Why hadn't I thought of this before? I could have them come every couple of weeks, and that part of the nightmare would be gone.

Two women and a man arrived promptly at ten. I had explained Nick's situation to the man on the phone, that the first visit would require a "deep cleaning."

"Oh, don't you worry," he said. "We've seen *everything*. My people will take good care of you."

They brought their own vacuum and all the supplies you could imagine. Standing in the living room, I saw them exchange pointed looks. I started getting nervous and switched into garrulous mode.

"Yes, so this is the living room slash bedroom. You can see he's a, uh, smoker." All five of us stared at the mountain of butts on his night table like we were in a museum. "Yep. That's for sure," I babbled. "I know it's pretty bad in here, but that's why I had them send three of you." My voice slid up into the high registers at the end of every sentence. Nick just stood there, like it was someone else's life.

In the corner of the kitchen was the trash can, which had overflowed to become just a pile of garbage. Every utensil, dish, and pot were tangled together in a foul sculpture decaying in the sink. At the same instant, we all looked at the refrigerator, but no one said a word.

"Oh, here, I've gotten a big box of trash bags." I smiled weakly. "I guess *they'll* get filled up, ha, ha!" By then I'm sure I, too, had the crazy eyes. The box slipped out of my flailing hand and crashed onto the pile of refuse. On impact, a million cockroaches of all sizes scurried out in every direction. That was it. The workers burst into a frantic three-way argument in Spanish. I tried to follow, but I couldn't. It didn't matter. I knew exactly what they were saying.

The man approached me. "I'm sorry, lady, but we cannot clean this. We are not allowed."

"What do you mean?" I asked. "It's just a few . . ." I didn't have the audacity to keep going.

"Missus, I see you have a big problem here. You know, there are companies that clean these situations. Hazardous materials and bugs. You should call them. I'm so sorry."

I could see that he truly was sorry. I watched them leave, along with all my high hopes, and then I looked into the kitchen. Now that the garbage mountain had been disturbed, it was roaches gone wild. And there he was, my crazy son, just leaning against the counter. La-di-da. I realized I was clenching my jaw like it held the rope that would save me from falling into the abyss.

"THAT'S IT! Do you know what just happened, Nick? The cleaning people, the people who CLEAN for a living, just left because this place is so disgusting," I screamed. "Do you understand what I'm saying? You live in such a filthy, foul way, you scared off the professionals! They said I have to call the hazmat team! The ones who clean up after murders and nuclear accidents! I can only imagine what *that* costs." I started crying. Nick looked at me with a stranger's indifference.

"Okay. You know what? You know what, buddy boy, WE'RE GONNA CLEAN THIS PLACE! That's right, you and me. You did this, and you're going to help me undo it."

I dragged him to the store with me, and we bought the necessary supplies. It was ninety degrees out that day. Of course it was.

Back home, we got on it. By "we," I mean I scurried around in boxer shorts and a tank top, bellowing at him, while he moved in slow motion holding open a big black trash bag. I sprayed the whole place with several cans of roach killer. It was like a cartoon—they kept emerging, seemingly coming from the bowels of the earth, the living ones scrambling over the bodies of the dead ones. Eventually I just donned gloves and just started scooping them up. Alive, dead, I didn't care; I just kept collecting roaches and filling bags.

"Look at this, Nick! This is really unbelievable. Do you think this is why I became a mother? Open that bag! No. Hold it OPEN. I can't get them in there if you don't give me the widest opening. Why do I have to keep telling you that? Imagine how proud I must feel right now. So very proud." I was drenched in sweat and sarcasm, yammering on incoherently. At one point, I looked up at Nick, and he was laughing to himself.

"Oh, this is *funny*? You find this situation amusing, do you? Well, I'll tell you what. Once this place is clean, you are not keeping food here anymore. That's right. No more dinners. No more shopping. No more food for you!" I declared. Realizing the absurdity of that, I added, "You are just going to have to spend your money and go eat elsewhere or eat at our house. You are not allowed to have food in your apartment." It occurred to me that poor Dee was going to be the real loser here. No food for Nick meant no food for her.

We spent a long time bringing bags to the dumpsters. Nick bumbled along, did what I told him, but seemed removed from what was happening. I returned the next day, banished Nick to the streets, and let off about ten roach bombs in the apartment. Six hours later I returned, opened the windows, and turned on the grimy fan. I tied a scarf around my nose and mouth and set about collecting roach carcasses with a dustpan and a yellow-gloved palm as Nick held the trash bag. Finally, the place seemed acceptable for a normal cleaning crew. I ended up establishing a yearslong business relationship with a fast-talking Russian who sent legions of house cleaners to the farthest corners of Los Angeles. We never met in person, but, somehow, I felt he knew me well.

One of the features of schizophrenia is the individual's decreased attention to personal cleanliness. In our case, we were blessed by a sprinkling of OCD that made Nick preoccupied with germs and such. Hard to believe that the occupant of the previously described abode worried about germs, but when it came to his body, he was scrupulously clean. I have no explanation for this at all. It is just his particular crazy. His fingernails were clipped and white. He washed his hair and shaved. He put his sleeve over his hand before touching a doorknob. The dichotomy was confounding. One day I realized that we hadn't bought toothpaste in what seemed like forever. I wondered if he even brushed his teeth. He assured me he did. I bought him toothpaste, but who the hell knew?

Every three weeks, we went faithfully to see Dr. Amiri. He tinkered with and adjusted the treatment, and eventually brought Nick to a place of stability we hadn't seen in years.

I drove by Dee's spot one day to explain why I wasn't coming by anymore. I gave her some money.

"So, Dee, why do you stay here? Do you like it?"

"It's a good spot," she said. "I feel safe here."

"What about a shelter or something? We could look around."

Dee flinched and jerked her right shoulder away from me. For a second her eyes were alight with something, but then it was gone. "No shelters. They aren't safe. People hurt each other in the shelters. Just like my dad."

"Your dad?"

"Yeah. He hurt himself. I was sitting at the kitchen table, eating an egg salad sandwich. He got mad at my ma, and then he went out on the porch and shot himself in the head. What a mess."

I gave her some more money and promised I'd stop by again. I did it pretty regularly for a while, and then I didn't. One day I passed her spot and she was not there. It appeared she'd gone.

I had arrived home with a bag of Nick's laundry. I knew that if I didn't do it, he would wear dirty clothes. When I dumped it on the floor, a bunch of cockroaches came out. Craig happened to be standing there.

"All it takes is ONE cockroach, Mimi. One." If he only knew. I hadn't told anyone about Nick's apartment. I felt such a jumble of shame and disgust about it that I just handled it alone.

"Okayokayokay! I get it. I know. I don't want them in the house either. I'll make sure."

"Oh really? And how are you going to do that?"

"Don't worry about it. I'll figure it out. You won't see a single cockroach."

That was how the parking lot system began. The lot at the Rite Aid near Nick was fairly empty most afternoons. A car would pull in now and then, but even in the bright, sunny light it felt secluded. Nobody knew me there, not like in Larchmont Village. I opened the door of my truck and pulled out a big black trash bag. Sauntering to the back of my vehicle as best I could with the unwieldy bundle, I leaned against the bumper. Nothing to see here. Move along.

I opened the bag and dumped all of the laundry onto the blacktop. A lone cockroach scurried into the perfectly designed flower bed nearby. Shaking the bag rigorously, I turned it inside out and shook again. Picking up the clothing piece by piece, I jerked each one back and forth to check for more insects. It had to be meticulously done—not one of them could be allowed to get through. His clothes smelled like cigarettes and sweat. Shaking a large towel, I saw three or four of them scurry off. Motherfuckers. A maybe-homeless lady walked by without even giving me a glance.

Brooke and I were sitting on her front steps. She lived directly around the corner from me. I could walk over there, get some love, and walk home in the space of an hour. She'd told me about a neighbor couple of hers. Both of them were architects. They had a son and a daughter. A good family. The daughter had gotten mixed up with some boy and became entrenched in gang life, addicted to heroin. The family was in shambles.

"I saw Diane this morning," Brooke said.

"Oh. How's it going with the daughter?" I asked.

"Not good. They've tried everything, but she won't leave the boyfriend. They begged her to go to rehab, but she refuses."

"How do these things happen? You think you're good parents, but that doesn't seem to matter."

"You know what she said to me? It was so sad."

"What?" I asked, not sure I wanted to know.

"She said that she has a fantasy that she just gets a gun and murders the boyfriend. She'd get the death penalty and be out of her misery, and her daughter would be freed from him and have a chance at recovery. Problem solved."

"Jesus, that is sad. But if it's a fantasy, why doesn't she just fantasize that her daughter comes home and gets better?" We both giggled guiltily. "You want to know what mine is?"

"Sure."

"I put Nick in the car with me and we drive off a cliff, Thelma and Louise style. Problem solved. I'm out of my misery and so is Nick. No more punching walls."

"Oh, dear," Brooke exhaled.

"Yeah, but the problem is the girls. It would wreck them forever. Otherwise I swear I would have done it already." I don't know if that was true, but it felt true. For a moment we just looked at each other, and the swath of maternal pretending fell away. We sat with the truth of what it means to be a mother.

"Let's have a coffee," Brooke said.

"Good idea."

I asked Dr. Amiri if he would like to see the writing I'd found. Nick was outside, smoking.

"Of course," he replied. "Any insight into his mind will be helpful."

I opened a notebook from Nick's kitchen counter and read the first entry out loud:

> I will conclude that my Judaism will die with my mother. She is an example of used chewing tobacco.

This, written in the scratchy, unhinged cursive of my son.

> As a boy, I was a wildflower, I went into awkward adolescence and started using magic potions to simulate the wildflower effect . . . This led to unconscious self-destruction eventually becoming very, very conscious. In retrospect, I see that I wasn't really my most balanced version of myself throughout all of this.

"No kidding," I said, softly, and handed him the notebook.

> Women are subject to 5% more water (read Newton) making them more vulnerable to different gravitas. Can't we drain them?

"That's fascinating," he said, and then continued reading out loud.

> Evil spirits whisper whisker ways,
> gray and sore muscles spasm with pulse
> and cripple dependents.

Chamomile sheepskin quilts.
Honey, there's someone in my brain.

To see the unspooling of your son's mind, like fine, wiry thread dancing away into blackness. To be able to identify the moment in time that it was written and compare realities. I realized then that my boy had *always* been leaving us; we just didn't know it.

I excused myself and went outside. The parking lot was empty of cars, and the cracked asphalt looked like a view of the earth from very far away. The weeds poking through had small yellow flowers. Nick stood with his back to me.

"Hey, Boyo, I need to tell you something."

As he turned, I thought I saw light falling off of him, scattering to the ground.

"You have schizophrenia. That's what you have. It's not any of the other things. It's schizophrenia."

He stood there, chin raised slightly, looking to the horizon like a sailor waiting for a sea change.

10

DIRT GRASS LIFE

As we settled into a period of relative calm with Nick, I realized I was dead. Not actually dead, of course, but just functioning. Barely. Keeping the big machine moving was all I did. That and trying to save Rose from the malaise that enveloped her. But as I turned to my youngest, I found I had nothing to give. I could fulfill surface quotidian wants for her—clothes or lessons or a ride to a concert—but a corpse offers poor hope of rejuvenating others.

One day I wandered into our local, funky yoga studio. It had housed classes for thirty years, long before yoga was hip. *At least it's close and cheap*, I thought, *and I'll get some exercise. That might help me.*

I went three times a week and studied with a beautiful, wise girl named Carmen. One day, I found myself doing a balance pose that had previously been impossible. It was no big deal, but as I stood there, I swelled with comfort at this thought: *I can't save Nick, but I can do this. Right now, I can stand balancing on one leg, and that's not nothing.*

Going into the practice of yoga in such a depleted state resulted in a shift that never would have been possible in my younger, more confident days. I was a wreck of a woman unrolling my brand-new, odd-smelling mat that first day. But I had a lot of open space inside, space previously filled up with hard-line ideas and opinions.

I kept going a few days a week and then every day. The girls who taught the poses also brought a lot of theory and philosophy to class—things I had scoffed at most of my life as hippy-dippy nonsense. I had a mental running commentary going most of the time.

Oh great, I'm next to Sweaty Guy again. I had names for all of them. Underpants Girl, BO Boy, Show-Off, Thumper. It was a regular stand-up comedy routine in my head. The perfect, thirtysomething teacher would say, "Stand tall. Let your chests be buoyant!" I'd think, *My chest hasn't been buoyant since I finished nursing Rose in '95!*

I cracked myself up.

One afternoon, I sat up from a pose to see a coin-sized pool of sweat on my mat right where the exact center of my forehead had been. It glistened. I could see lines, like ancient cave paintings, colors reflected that weren't even in the room. *It's a fingerprint of my brain,* I thought. *A perfect representation of everything inside.*

I started listening to what the teachers were saying.

Standing in the front of the room by the window, my feet flat against the floor, I was aware of both surfaces, skin and wood. I could feel my legs, my spine, straight and dependable, holding the skull that cradled my mind. Carmen's words entered my cochlea, gently moving the tiny hair cells with their vibrations.

"Truth is the same always," she said, quoting the sutras.

Outside the window the city moved into evening.

The next week, my friend Jill dragged me to a meditation class with a world-renowned teacher. I was skeptical. I can't even sit still for a TV show, so the idea of looking inward for twenty silent minutes was terrifying. Bliss Consciousness? The red wine was working quite well for me, thank you very much.

Nothing in my head. Is it possible? Well, not nothing, because I am thinking this. Go to the mantra, like he said. Am I thinking? I don't know. Remember, the mantra is the most charming, go there. Okay, okay . . . Eventually, nothingness.

I liked it. It turns out that sitting in a chair with your eyes closed for twenty minutes twice a day changes something inside of you. One day, walking to Brooke's house, I thought, *I'm going barefoot. When was the last time I walked barefoot in the city?* I set out with the single intention of noticing what the different surfaces felt like on the soles of my feet. Grass. Dirt. Sidewalk. Asphalt. I wanted to be in the moment, like I had been taught. It wasn't a complex exercise at all, but for me, it marked my return to the world of the living.

Dirt. Grass. Life.

All this coincided with the terrible adolescence of Rose Amelia O'Rourke. My new, spiritual self awakened to be greeted with scorn. She hated the way I chewed my food. She thought I was stupid. I tapped the steering wheel to music in a manner that deserved the death penalty. I danced around like a circus animal, trying to elicit a smile, only to receive an iron stare and contemptuous silence. *Okay,* the new me decided, *I've learned that being reactive only makes things worse. I am going to continue to douse her with buckets full of love until she is soothed.*

"I hate you," she would scream.

"Well, I love you," I'd say, feigning calm.

"I fucking HATE you," she'd scream louder.

"I love you sooooooo much," I'd respond.

I could do it forever.

She made some neighborhood friends and was having a social life. Now that I felt stronger, more alive, all I wanted was to make her happy. If rejecting me and hanging with her friends was what she needed, fine.

Yes, I was still angry as hell that Nick was sick. I still drank way too much wine. I was still in denial about what this was doing to my marriage, my family. But I did have moments of peace and acceptance.

"I'm going to Jeremy's tonight with Shannon to watch some movies," Rose announced.

Oh, this is good, she's having fun.

"Shannon's dad will drive me home."

It was about ten thirty when my phone rang. I had poured a

tumbler of wine by then, alone at home preparing for a descent into television and self-pity. Craig was in Washington.

"Mom." Lucy, calling from Santa Cruz, was crying.

"Lucy! What is it?"

"Shannon just called. She said that Rose drank a bunch of vodka and passed out, and they don't know what to do," she wailed.

"Wait. What? She's just around the corner at Jeremy's. His grand-father is there watching them."

"Well, go over there!"

I glanced longingly at my untouched wine and then ran down to the car. I pounded on the door until Shannon answered.

"Where is she?"

"Uh, upstairs . . ." Shannon and her cohorts stood before me, a cluster of inebriated dunces. Where the hell was the grandfather?

I ran up and into an empty bedroom. "Where is she?" I yelled to them. I could hear water running. Someone muttered, "In the bathroom." As they bumped comically into each other behind me, I saw my youngest daughter lying akimbo in the bathtub. Her jeans were down around her ankles, shoes on, eyes open, with cold water running on her head from the shower. It looked like a rape scene. She was out cold.

"What the hell happened here?" I kneeled next to the tub and tried to shake her awake.

"We think she might have, like, drunk too much alcohol or something," someone said.

"Ya think?" I shrieked. "Why are her pants down? What did you do to her?" There had been a couple of sketchy incidents in the neighborhood of a sexual nature, boys taking advantage of drunk girls. All the parents were on edge.

"No, no. Nothing like that," Shannon said. "I wanted to get her in the shower and I tried to take her pants off, so they wouldn't get wet. I couldn't get them over her shoes."

Only then did I turn around and see the grandfather standing sheepishly behind the kids.

"Where were you? How did you let this happen?" I yelled.

I don't know if it was a language thing—he was Greek—but I never got a coherent sentence out of him. Just then, Shannon's father arrived to pick them up. Rose started to moan and move a bit, so I knew she was, at the very least, alive. First, we had to get her pants up.

"Shannon, get over here and help me." That was a bumbling mess, those damn skinny jeans.

"Wait, Mimi! I have to find her belt. She needs her belt!" Everyone started looking for the belt.

"We got a dime holding up a dollar here," I yelled. "FORGET THE BELT."

In the movies, you see men scoop up passed-out women and sweep them to safety with relative ease. Well, I'm here to tell you that's not how it goes. She was little and skinny, and I was quite strong from all the yoga, but what unfolded was a ridiculous dance that brought to mind trying to stuff slippery spaghetti into a ziplock bag. She was all arms and legs and seemed to weigh a thousand pounds. At one point, as I was drag-carrying her across the bedroom, I glowered at the two men who were just standing there, watching.

"A little HELP here, gentlemen?"

Shannon's dad, her grandfather, and I got Rose into my car. I took off as though getting away would solve everything.

I got Rose, semiconscious by then, into the house and onto the living room couch. Now what?

"Theresa, it's me. Something happened. Rose has alcohol poisoning, I think . . . I don't know what to do!"

"Hold on, darling. I'll be right there."

"What do I do? I don't know what to do. Do I let her sleep it off?" I asked when she arrived from across the street.

"No. We need to take her to the hospital," Theresa said. "I'll get my car and meet you in front."

When I think of that night, I am baffled by my own ineptness.

Why didn't I call 911? FOUR times I carried that girl. Once into my car. Then back into our house. Then out to Theresa's car. Finally, into the hospital, only to have her slither out of my hands, roll across the floor, and slam into a wall at the emergency room window. That was my crowning moment—all the late-night patients, the ones who are really messed up, were gawking at *me*. The lady behind the window, peering down at my inert child. The guard only barely, just enough for me to register, shaking his head from side to side.

"I think she may have had too much to drink," I said.

An orderly came and finally, movie-style, scooped her up and swept her away. Standing there under the fluorescent lighting, I felt unworthy. I sat in a plaid chair.

Eventually a nurse came to get me. Rose was still out like a light but now had an IV in her arm. She looked flat as a cardboard cutout on the bed. They told me that she had alcohol poisoning, would probably be okay, but all they could do was hydrate her and wait. It was going to be a long night. I called Lucy and told her not to worry.

Grinding my knuckles into my temples, I went to sit vigil, dreading calling Craig with this one.

Well, sitting vigil on a crappy metal chair sucks. I shifted and repositioned myself, but there was no comfort to be found—physically or emotionally.

Look at her. Sleeping peacefully, oblivious to all that's going on. Craig's up in Washington doing the same thing. Everything is going to hell, and I'm stuck on this shitty chair all night.

I stood up, looked around, took off my shoes, and crawled into the bed with Rose. At the very least, I was going to be warm and comfortable. I wrapped my body around her like I used to when she slept in our bed, taking note for a second, triumphantly, of how much she would hate that. I pretended we were at home and she was a baby.

There was no deceiving myself when I opened my eyes a few hours later. Oh, that wonderful second before the floodgates of consciousness open. Then, the deluge of facts came to take me down.

I am in a hospital bed with Rose. Is she awake? Will she recover? We were spooning, she in front of me. I rolled onto my back and stared at the water-stained acoustic ceiling. Rose stirred. She rolled over and looked at me. The room, the IV—she must have had a little fact-flood of her own. Her eyes welled up with tears in that dramatic way that young children cry, so quickly, so completely.

"Do you hate me?" Rose asked.

"Oh, Rose, of course I don't hate you," I murmured. "I love you. I'll always love you."

"What happened?"

I gave her a somewhat sanitized version. She was so scared, I couldn't be mad. The doctor arrived to take a look; she was fine and could be discharged. We got the requisite lecture on the perils of juvenile drinking and left with lots of colorful pamphlets.

Once outside, I remembered I had no car. It was 6:00 a.m. on Sunday morning. I couldn't bring myself to call a friend because my life was just too ridiculous. I called a taxi. Soon, a big Romanian man in a beat-up cab pulled up, spit out his window, and asked, "You call cab?"

We gingerly got into the foul vehicle. Rose was wrapped in a hospital blanket, and I was too grateful to be walking out with my daughter alive to be mortified about the fact that I was wearing my pajamas. As soon as the vehicle began to move, Rose started retching. I smoothed her forehead and told her to hang on, we'd be home in a minute.

"What is happening? She still sick?" the cabbie barked. "No vomit in cab!"

Are you sure about that? I thought, surveying the interior. "Oh, she's fine, let's just get her home."

"I pull over!"

Despite my protests, Romanian Guy pulled over, and Rose vomited into the gutter. He beamed at me. "You see, I know these things." He wasn't beaming when we pulled up to our house after he had stopped for two more gutter barfings.

We stared icily at each other as we completed our transaction. Then I turned on my heels and walked away without so much as a thank you. I showed him. My newfound enlightenment was fading rapidly.

Once inside, I cleaned Rose up and put her to bed, then got into mine. I had to call Craig. I knew this was going to be a particularly rough one for him. He had done the hardest thing—he'd quit drinking—but now he lived in fear of the kids having the gene for alcoholism and addiction. I burrowed deeper into the bedding and stared at my phone.

The genetics. What, exactly, is our responsibility for our genetics? Who do we blame?

When Craig and I first moved into Larchmont Village, a couple of scrappy artists from a downtown loft, all I wanted was to fit into the life there. These days my so-called good address was starting to seem like a bad joke. My family was a spectacle. The idea of being a respectable family was all facade, rapidly crumbling.

The light filtered in, creating a parade of shadows for me to watch, each holding an event, a loss, a betrayal. I had worked so hard to get Nick to a place of just neutral, not even *better*, and now I was just beginning to see the damage done to Rose.

I got out of bed and went into my studio. *Perhaps I'll paint for a while and drink some vodka myself. Maybe I will paint my own* Guernica. *Then I'll call Craig. Eventually, I'll sleep.*

I got as far as the paint and the vodka.

When I woke up the next morning, I called Craig and told him. In the silence that followed, I could hear the shattering of something complicated and fragile. Then he began to cry.

Nick was twenty-two now and fairly stable on his meds. I was working on getting him into a genome study on schizophrenia at the National Institute of Mental Health in DC. I had an elaborate plan to get him there under that guise and then convince him to stay for another more comprehensive study. The application process was long and arduous; it would be eight months before we'd know if he was selected.

Every so often I'd arrive at his apartment with art supplies and set up his breakfast nook as a studio. The paints and brushes would sit there, rot away, and eventually end up in the trash. I didn't even know where all his old paintings were.

He liked to go with me on errands, get out and around. He'd sit quietly in the passenger seat as I rambled.

"Do you love me, Nick?"

No answer.

"Do you love anyone?"

Nothing.

"Nick! What about your sisters? What if Lucy died? Would you even care?"

"Sure," he'd say in exactly the same tone as when I asked if he wanted lunch.

We were driving down Norton, and a guy cut me off. I swore at him. When we reached Sixth Street it was impossible to get across, and no one would let me pass. I went into a tirade. Just as we got to Wilshire, another driver cut me off.

"Son of a bitch! What the hell is wrong with these people? Does anyone know how to drive? I hate them all." We sat at the red light with the echo of my outburst reverberating in the car. I was breathing hard. I looked over at Nick, who had not spoken in two hours, and our eyes met.

"How's that meditation working out for you, Ma?" he asked.

It was book club night. We were a group of smart, funny, irreverent loudmouths who had been together for many years. We'd found each other amidst the manicured lawns of Larchmont Village. I threw together a salad, grabbed the book, and walked down the street. At our club, we actually talked about the books—discussions that would lead us into many subjects like politics, art, and philosophy, which could devolve into debate, altercations, and hilarity. We were also very good friends, so the subject matter usually became personal at the beginning and the end of most meetings.

That night, I had to get home because I was nervous about what might happen with me gone. Nick was at the house. I asked the hostess where the Saran Wrap was. Opening the drawer, I stood in wonder. There were neatly lined-up boxes of foil, cellophane, wax paper, ziplock bags—not a thing out of place. In my house, that drawer is always a holy mess. Nobody puts anything back correctly. The boxes are open, weird vegetable bags are stuffed in, crumpled brown lunch bags everywhere. Every metal twist tie from every box of bags I've ever bought is tangled in the bottom. Looking at this tidy drawer, I saw the perfect example of a managed life. A regular family. My drawer just screamed *nuthouse!*

Although I was anxious, I walked home slowly, reluctant to leave the cocoon of normalcy at my neighbor's.

I spent most of my time contending with small catastrophes and trying to love Rose into happiness. It wasn't working. She stopped even trying in school, and wouldn't that be the final indicator of my failure as a mother? What future would she have without a high school diploma? Thanks to yoga, I was now able to do a handstand in the middle of the room, but I couldn't seem to get my family on track. With a crazy son, an angry daughter, and an absent husband, life was an endless game of Whac-A-Mole.

"I'm a vegetarian now," Rose announced as she walked into the kitchen. I looked down at the large chuck roast I'd just put on the counter. *Great.*

"Oh, that's nice," I said. "That can be healthy. You just have to be very careful to get all the nutrients you need."

"Oh really? You think I don't know that?"

"No, Rose, I don't think you don't know that. I just wanted to say that I knew that. I mean, you know . . . oh, never mind. Just let me know what you want me to get. Put it on the list."

And the battle for the kitchen began. The one place that had always been my domain was under siege, my hands tied by my vow to make everything up to her. I was screwed.

"Mom, that is so unhealthy. I can't believe you eat that and want to feed us that. It's disgusting."

A cheeseburger?

"It's good, Ma," said Nick, who'd shown up for dinner.

"Oh great. That's right, you're probably making him worse," she said as she flounced out of the room with smoldering disdain.

Derelict in my duties once again, I nonetheless joined Nick at the table for cheeseburgers.

As the weeks progressed, she moved from being a vegetarian to being vegan, getting rather thin and pale. She refused to discuss it. "The List" was getting scary expensive. I found myself buying one-inch square brownish bars from the health food store that cost $7.99.

Massages appeared to improve her disposition, so off we went to the Korean spa! Unheard of vitamins? Sure. Outlandishly expensive herbs and teas? Absolutely. A super weird chiropractor in Venice Beach whose office looked like a front for drug dealers? No problem. I was spending my entire weekly budget on Rose. After promising Craig I wouldn't, I even let her bring home a stray dog. She swore she'd find him a home. The next day she named him Woody. *Good move, Feldy.*

Rose's schoolwork was not improving. So I got involved— way too involved. I found myself keeping track of her assignments, dogging her to finish them.

"Just get it written, and I'll edit it for you, Rose."

If she was late or forgot something, I'd run to the school. If she called during the day and begged me to come take her out of school because she was too depressed, I did it. The "editing" eventually led to me writing the actual papers. I was out of control. I couldn't lose another child.

"Oh, this is good, Rose. One of the books on your list is the one we're reading this month in book club. I'll *really* be able to help you with that." Yes, I actually said that with a straight face.

I wrote a six-page essay, from beginning to end, on the caste system in India and how it reflected other social structures throughout the world. It was actually very interesting. I did a lot of research. One night it hit me: *Wait,* I thought. *We may have a problem. It's going to be obvious to the teacher that someone of superior intellect wrote this.* (That was the problem?) *I'd better dumb this down a bit so her teacher doesn't get suspicious.* I sat back and thought about it. *Actually, no. I'm going for it! Leave it as it is!*

Rose turned the paper in on a Friday. "When do you think we'll get it back?" I asked anxiously.

"I don't know, Mom. It takes a long time sometimes. Whatever."

A week went by. I was dying to see my grade. I began pestering Rose. She looked at me like the buffoon I was and walked out of the room.

The following Wednesday I asked her again. "Oh yeah, I got it back on Monday," she said. "I forgot."

She *forgot*? "Well, let me see it," I said as casually as I could.

I got a C. I could not believe my eyes. What was wrong with this charlatan who called himself a history teacher? What could possibly be wrong with my wonderful paper? Well, he was pretty articulate about what was wrong. There were plenty of comments in the margins, written in light-blue ink.

"This is ridiculous, Rose," I cried. "How could he give me, I mean, *this*, a C?"

"I don't care," she said.

"Well, I care! This is completely unfair. This is an A paper, to be sure. I'm going to make an appointment for a conference. He can't do this."

Rose didn't have to say a word. She just took the paper out of my hands. The "Did you hear what you just said?" was implicit.

"I'm totally losing it," I said to Brooke the next day over coffee. "I have become everything I hate. I am enabling Rose to completely slack off because I am so afraid of losing another child."

"What do you mean?"

"I am Rose's bitch. That is what I have become. I'm so afraid to add to her unhappiness that I will do literally anything." I confessed the tale of the essay.

"Mimi!" Brooke was laughing uncontrollably.

"I know. I know! I was actually going to go in there and confront him." I was laughing, too, by then. "I mean, that's not something I would do if *she'd* written the paper! Who am I? It just chaps my hide that the son of a bitch gave me a C!"

"Good thing you didn't dumb it down," Brooke said, smiling.

When I arrived home, the answering machine was blinking.

"Hello, this is the emergency room at Kaiser Sunset, and we have a John Doe here that we believe might be someone you know. Please call us back as soon as possible," the black box told me. It was 1:15 p.m. The message had come in at 9:45 a.m.

I sunk slowly into my desk chair. I listened to it again. In my panic, I kept thinking, *John Doe. Isn't that how they refer to dead bodies?*

"Hello, my name is Miriam Feldman, and I have a son who has schizophrenia. I received a message that there is a John Doe there who might . . . be . . . him?" My voice faltered.

It turned out that Nick had been sitting outside our neighborhood sandwich shop the afternoon before and had passed out on the pavement. A woman ran inside for help, and they called the paramedics.

He'd been taken to the hospital but had no identification. He woke up and told them our home number, then passed out again. No one knew why. He was in there for two days. He didn't remember anything. When we left, the nurse handed me a bag with his belongings. It consisted of a pack of cigarettes, a lighter, and his favorite "The Who" T-shirt that had been cut raggedly in half by the paramedics when they tried to revive him.

The scene played itself out in my mind as similar scenes I had seen on television: The paramedics have the inert patient on a gurney. He is not breathing. They take out the oddly shaped medical scissors and urgently chop, chop, chop the shirt to access the chest. The shirt is pulled out from under him and thrown aside. It turns out someone retrieves it and returns it. I still have that shirt in a ziplock bag at the back of my drawer today, with the Bob Dylan one.

I just couldn't get over the John Doe thing. I was more shaken up by the idea that he'd been called a "John Doe" than by the fact that he'd passed out. A John Doe? He wasn't that. He wasn't some unknown, uncared-for nobody. He was Nick Fucking O'Rourke.

I went to the shop to find out what had happened. Nick had gotten a sandwich and was outside eating when the woman came in and said he'd gone unconscious. She'd sat on the ground with him until the ambulance arrived, lifting his head off the sidewalk onto her lap.

I tracked her down and called her. I cried (of course) and thanked her for holding his head.

One thing was certain: we had to find a way to make sure Nick had identification on him at all times. I drove to Petco. I walked up to the arcade-style machine and inserted some coins. I left the store with two dog-bone shaped metal tags with our phone number on them. One for Woody, who was clearly our dog now. And one for Nick, which I put on his wrist.

Rose had graduated from veganism to the Gut Diet, introduced by her latest boyfriend. When just the week before it had seemed the next logical step would be simply grazing on the backyard lawn, she suddenly started bringing boxes of meat and bones into the house.

There was a large bucket filled with chicken feet. Steaming caul-drons sat for days on the stove. I entered the kitchen one day to find a good-looking, curly-headed kid surveying my refrigerator.

"Oh, hi. Are you Rose's mom? I'm Isaac," he said pleasantly.

Isaac. "Jew?" I asked.

Rose appeared just in time to hear that and give me a withering stare.

"Um, yes, I'm Jewish," he said.

"Nice," I said. Rose actually stomped her foot.

"Yeah," said Isaac. "My grandfather is a rabbi."

"Really? How interesting," I cooed. "I think I'll just call you by your Hebrew name, Yitzchak." I used my most guttural Hebrew pronunciation. By that point I had realized Rose was going to hate me no matter what I did. What the hell? I'd lost control of my kitchen. The dogs ruled the yard. Nick had just informed me he was thinking of going off his meds. So, from time to time, I allowed myself a little fun.

Like a biblical torrent of plagues, things kept happening to Rose. She had a bicycle accident and broke her arm. It was shattered in a way that required surgery and a track of metal staples to close the wound. Then she developed a cyst on her upper thigh. We went to the doctor and were informed it should be removed. It would be an outpatient procedure and require careful tending to afterward.

Every day after school, Rose would lie on the bathroom floor and I'd change the dressing. My job was to ever so slowly pull the slimy, gooey gauze out of her leg while she screamed into a towel. That was the easy part. Then I had to carefully refill the opening with new packing. I even had a special little tool for doing it. The problem was the gauze liked to just pop right back out as soon as you made any progress, and then you had to start all over. It was such an under-taking—considering Rose's pain, my queasiness, the uncomfortable location of the wound itself (right below her crotch)—that the two of us became unhinged every time we had to do it. She'd scream in pain,

I'd scream because she was screaming, and intermittently we'd both laugh hysterically.

"Ew . . . ooh . . . Rose, look at this, it's disgusting." I'd hold up a drippy piece.

"Noooo," she'd yell into the towel she kept over her face in order to pretend she wasn't actually there.

It was in the confines of the kids' bathroom that Rose and I cemented our bond. The subway tiles Craig had painstakingly placed in perfect lines gleamed. He'd painted the walls Gilded Trip, a barely yellow color. It glowed. Vintage embroidered curtains I'd made out of a tablecloth hung above us like a banner. I remembered my hands rubbing cotton towels over wet baby heads, soft skin of children dripping wet. It was in that room, surrounded by ointments and gauze, that I proved there was nothing I wouldn't do for her.

Nick continued to take his medication. There hadn't been any holes in the walls in a while. He'd settled into a peaceful, if vacant, routine. I was still working on the NIMH study, and the lady over there was encouraging. Craig would be home soon for the fall months, and I was looking forward to his return. At that point, it was beginning to feel like our marriage was just a long telephone call.

Nick was accompanying me on a day of errands. I had to go to the valley, where we could go to one of his favorite lunch spots. He was fairly silent that day, so I filled the space with my incessant chatter.

"Nick. Look at those pants. Can you believe it? What is she thinking?" We were at a stoplight watching pedestrians. No response.

"Whew, look at him. He's a rough stretch of highway. Look at those feet." Nothing.

I could go on all day like that. He was alive. He was with me. It felt like treading water with my son in tow; maybe we weren't getting anywhere, but we weren't sinking either.

"Hey, Mom, isn't this where you turn for Todai Buffet? I think it's up about two blocks on the left." Suddenly he was present.

We pulled in to the parking lot and got out of the car. "Holy moly, it's hot out here," I said. "The old Indian summer, it'll get you every time. It's as hot as it was in Israel." I just couldn't shut up.

Once inside the air-conditioned restaurant, we loaded our plates with sushi and an array of Asian delicacies. Just as we sat down, a man came up to our table.

"Excuse me," he said, "are you the driver of a gray Toyota?"

"Yes," I said. Now what?

"Well, I want you to know that when you opened your door, you slammed it into my car," he said in a flat tone.

"Oh, I'm so sorry. Was there any damage?"

"That's beside the point," he said. "You shouldn't just bang into other people's cars."

"Would you like me to go look at it with you? If there is any damage, I will of course take care of it," I offered.

"Yes, let's do that."

I looked at Nick. "Just stay here, hold our table, and watch my purse. I'll be right back."

We walked through the big restaurant and out into the heat. There was no damage. This was some kind of macho "teach-a-lesson" thing. As we stood there having the absurd conversation he seemed hell-bent on, I felt a presence behind me. I turned my head and squinted into the sun and realized it was Nick.

"Nick! What are you doing here?" I asked harshly. "I *told* you to stay at the table! Where's my purse? Did you leave my purse?"

He didn't say anything but strategically moved between me and the man. The man said, "Well, fine. It looks like there is no damage. I just think you should be more careful in the future." He got into his car, and Nick and I walked back across the scorching asphalt.

"Nick. What the hell? Can't you just do what I tell you? Now they might have cleared our table. And you left my purse! Why would you do that?" On and on I went.

Quietly, Nick said, "I didn't like the way he was talking to you."

We went inside and sat down. My purse was fine. It dawned on me: he had been protecting me. He had perceived a threat and made the decision to disregard my instructions because he cared about me. He was not going to let his mother be in peril. His mind may not be fully functioning, but he had a heart, and it was a good heart.

He wasn't gone.

11

THE CERTAINTY OF
GLASS TO PAVEMENT

It was 2010, and Nick was twenty-five years old. Craig came back just in time for Halloween, which was an extravaganza in our neighborhood. People loaded their kids into cars and drove from all around Los Angeles. Buster always went nuts, and now we had Woody ratcheting everything up. Craig was sore at me for letting Rose get another dog, and I spent a lot of time running interference. I cleaned things up before anyone saw them, replaced broken and chewed items. Nothing had changed for me; it was just the canine version of the game.

"Mimi, I'm concerned about your dogs tomorrow night. How are you going to deal with this?" Craig asked me. Note: *your* dogs. Yes, they had become *my* problem, both of them. I started searching the internet. I remembered the bottle of Valium Dr. Amiri had prescribed Nick for occasional use.

"Is it safe to give a dog . . ." I typed into the computer. Wow, in second place "Valium" popped up. I wasn't the only maniac in the world. It appeared that it was fine.

No one was in the kitchen on Halloween night. I took out two slices of bread and buttered them liberally. I was lining up the allowed number of pills in the butter when my neighbor came in.

"What are you doing, Meems?"

There was no way to go with this one but the truth.

"Okay. Craig is still furious with me about Woody, and of course Rose isn't here to help. Those dogs are gonna go nuts out there tonight, so I looked it up on the internet, and it said I can give them Valium. These are Valium. Nick's Valium. I'm giving it to my dogs. It's going to keep them calm," I said. There it was. The whole ugly truth.

"You can't do that!" she whisper-yelled. Oh, great, I didn't know she was one of those dog people. I was about to be shamed, big time.

"That is a complete waste! Give me some of those," she cackled.

We stood at my butcher-block island and picked six of the tablets out of the sandwiches. We didn't even need water to take them; the butter made it easy. We tiptoed out and gave the rest to the dogs. It was a peaceful Halloween.

Like I said, I'm not proud of it, but it happened.

Our house in Washington was burglarized the week before Thanksgiving. A neighbor called and told us the front door was wide open and the place had been ransacked. Craig had to go up there. It was a rather sorry robbery; there wasn't much of anything with any worth up there. Craig's computer was gone, and one of the big, old-style televisions. The other one had been left in the yard, as though the burglar had decided it wasn't worth its weight in anything. I'd always teased Craig about his obsession about locking things up, but this time it had worked. Before he'd left he put anything of value in the barn, which he'd transformed into Fort Knox. He constructed old-timey security: big logs of wood that fit into brackets to secure doors, padlocks upon padlocks. With the insurance, we actually came out ahead.

The sad thing about the event was that they took Craig's vintage Leatherman knife, which had been a birthday gift from Nick. Craig never took it off his belt, except when he flew. He'd left it on the kitchen table before going to the airport. It was the talisman that held the boy who was lost to him.

When I told Nick what had happened, he immediately responded, "That's great! Now we know what I can get Dad for Christmas."

Another aspect of Nick's manifestation of schizophrenia was his seemingly endless optimism. It made no sense. That was definitely not an identified feature of the disease. Occasionally, I would complain to him about one of his sisters as we drove around the city. I'd describe some slight they'd committed or express hurt feelings, and he'd always respond with something like "Oh, I don't think she meant that. Maybe she just was having a bad day."

He had also become very puritanical about the girls. Lucy's outgoing message on her phone says: "Hello, it's Lucy, leave me something juicy!" He expressed concern that this greeting was a bit risqué and suggested I talk to her about it. He admonished me to make sure that their attire was appropriate. He was concerned about the boys they hung out with. I had no idea about Nick's sexuality. It seemed to have gone dormant. I had already seen so many things a mother shouldn't have to that I couldn't let my mind go there.

"You know, Craig, if Nick *had* to get schizophrenia, at least he seems to have gotten the good schizophrenia," I said one night on the front porch.

"Really?" he asked. "What exactly do you mean by that?"

"Well. Think about all the people you see on the street corners. They're a mess. They seem tortured and angry, hollering at things that aren't there. At least he's not like that."

"So he has the genteel strain of schizophrenia." Craig smiled.

"Yeah, and don't forget the OCD. That's a blessing. At least he keeps himself clean. With most people that is a big, big problem."

"I don't even begin to get it. Sometimes I think he's just lazy. I mean, he sleeps late every single day. That's a big problem."

"What, he's going to miss the board meeting?"

I don't think Craig completely gets it, even now. Things are going on in Nick's head that we can't even get near. It's a whole other world.

We searched until we found a Leatherman knife like the one that had been stolen. Nick didn't generally give gifts anymore. On my birthday or Mother's Day, I would receive a piece of typing paper folded in half containing an inscription written with colored pencils. In his diligent cursive, the front would say: *Happy Mother's Day.* Inside: *Have A Nice Holiday. Sincerely, Nick.*

Christmastime rolled around, and it was a good one, colored lights and a big, fat tree. Scarlett and the family drove down in their huge Winnebago. Happy kids running all over the place. Lots of cooking. Lucy and Rose made their signature pies. On Christmas morning, we all convened at the tree to exchange gifts. We saved Nick's gift to his dad until last. I prompted him, and he went over to Craig and said, "Here, Dad. This is for you from me."

Craig fought back tears when he saw what it was.

"Look, Dad, it's just like the other one," Nick said with more emotion than I'd heard in years. All three girls and I were crying like big old babies, and for a minute everything was sweet and sad and perfect. Like a string of tiny white holiday lights, everything connected and lit up.

I was working on a mural in a backyard in West LA, painting bougainvillea on the pool-area walls. I painted flower after flower after flower; it was soothing and enjoyable. I was eating lunch when my phone rang. The lady from the National Institute of Mental Health said Nick had been accepted into the study! They would fly Craig, Nick, and me there in March, and the girls could participate whenever they wanted. For once I wasn't in a quandary about whether to call the old man.

"Craig! You won't believe it. I got Nick into the study. We're going to DC in March," I gushed.

"Well, aren't you something, Feldy," he said.

I knew this was going to be it. The thing that changed everything.

March rolled around, and we got Nick all packed and headed to the airport. I was giddy.

There was a huge, Craftsman-style residence lodge in a garden setting for the study participants. We arrived late on Saturday night, so we had Sunday to acclimate and prepare for the intake procedures on Monday. We were given a room with two queen-size beds for the three of us. Nick went to bed, exhausted. Craig and I played a raucous game of Scrabble. It was warm and cozy, and we were both optimistic for a change.

We were shocked seeing Nick's body. The medication had caused him to gain a lot of weight, but it was hidden from us by his ever-present sweatshirt. In this shared room, we saw his large belly and were taken aback. Who was this person? Craig and I slept fitfully in the eerie light as Nick, who had woken up, watched cartoons all night.

Monday morning, the breakfast room was bustling. Many guests had arrived the night before. A family sat at each table—mothers, fathers, and mostly teenagers or young adult kids. The food was served buffet style, filling the room with a steam of aromas.

While Nick was up getting his food, I said, "Hey, Craig. Look at these families. It's a genome study, so at each table one of them is the crazy one. Let's guess who!"

"It's pretty clear who it is at our table," Craig replied dryly.

"No, no, no, let's do it. It'll be fun. I have great craydar."

"Great what?"

"Craydar. You know, like gaydar, except for crazy people."

"Oh my God," he said, shaking his head slowly, just like Nick.

Thus, the parlor game Pick-A-Nut was born. We entertained ourselves stealthily the whole time we were there. It wasn't until our last day that I discovered something sobering while reading through a pile of paperwork. The NIMH is part of the larger National Institutes of Health, and it turned out that the residents of our guesthouse participated in studies throughout the center. It was one thing to indulge in gallows humor ourselves, but it then dawned on me that we were among people with cancer and other deadly diseases. Suddenly the game lost its luster. We had been wagering over who would live and who would die.

"Well, this isn't funny at all," I said to Craig, and showed him the pamphlet.

"Hey, it was your idea."

"Should have known there was nothing to laugh about," I said.

"If this week hasn't shown you that, I don't know what will."

I couldn't argue.

After breakfast on Monday, we'd gone to meet our contact person, Helen, a social worker. I had been talking to her by telephone for almost a year, so it felt like we were old friends. After introductions, she described the study. Our participation would be limited to brain scans and blood tests, but Nick's was much more involved. After our tests, we played board games until he was done.

"So, Nick, there's something Dad and I wanted to talk to you about," I began.

No response.

"There's another study here at the NIMH we thought you might want to consider."

He looked up.

"Yeah, Nick," Craig went on. "It's a longer-term one where you'd stay here for a while."

"Oh, I don't think I'd want that."

"Just wait and hear about it before you say that," I continued. "It's really interesting. You stay here, in this beautiful place, for a few months. The doctors slowly take you off all your medication, so you can stabilize under their care."

"It'd be a great way to see how you are now, buddy, after all these years," Craig said. It had been almost six years since the diagnosis of schizophrenia.

"Then they can reevaluate you and maybe find better medications."

Nick began to slowly shake his head.

"That's okay. Just think about it. Tomorrow we can go over and see the place and you can get a better idea."

We meandered back to the guesthouse, pointing out flowers and plants we liked along the way.

The next morning, we went to the long-term study building. It was incredible. They showed us all the facilities. Each patient had his or her own room. There was a gym and a recreation room with a television and games. They had their own cafeteria with a diet tailored to nurture the brain. They had art therapy and social activities, a basketball court. All the people who worked there had the bright positivity of those who believe in their work.

Oh, please, please, let him agree to stay, I prayed with all my might.

At dinner that night, we tried to make him see the opportunity that was being offered. He actually would have a new start. He'd be healthy and in shape and given the best medications available by world-class doctors. He agreed to go back and look again the next day, after his final MRIs.

I was sure he'd agree to stay. It could not be possible that I'd worked for a year, gotten him on an actual airplane, flown across our country, only to fail. Midmorning, the three of us made our way over there. Everything we looked at had the new green of spring, lit by the light of a March sun. We asked questions of nurses, doctors, residents. We ate lunch there to see how the food was. As we finished up, I asked, "So, Nick. What do you think about the other study?"

"No," he said clearly. "I want to go home."

It was over. Craig and I both knew better than to argue. It was only about two in the afternoon. We had planned to stay overnight, settle him in on Friday, and fly home after that. We returned to the guesthouse without another word.

"Let's just get the hell out of here," I said tonelessly to Craig as soon as we were alone. What was the point of staying another night? The place felt depressing and cold now. He got on the telephone to arrange things, and we were on our way to the airport by four thirty that afternoon.

We dropped Nick off at his dark apartment in Los Angeles. Once home, we walked silently in, Craig to the bedroom and me to my studio. I stuffed all the papers in a file marked NIMH and slammed the drawer like I was shooting a gun.

Lucy decided to do her last year of college at University of California at Riverside and moved back home. I was happy; it was pretty grim at the house back then, and Lucy brought light with her. She was at school most of the weekdays and had a boyfriend in Santa Barbara, so we didn't see her much. But just having her home tempered the *Psycho* component of my relationship with Rose. Over the past two years, Rose and I had become like a tangle of roots growing in a confined space, all twisted and confused. It wasn't getting better.

Nick's dental situation had been lurking in the sidelines for a while. I'd opened a drawer in his kitchen and found every toothbrush and tube of toothpaste I'd ever bought jammed in there.

"What the what, Nick?" I started out yelling this time. "Do you ever brush your teeth?"

"Sure, yeah I do," he mumbled.

"Oh, REALLY, you do? Then how do you explain all this?"

Silence.

By then I had deduced that Nick had a bizarre hygiene regime consisting of Simple Green, paper towels, Ivory soap, and a very expensive brand of shampoo. He kept himself clean-shaven with an electric shaver. Beyond that lay a field of imagination I didn't want to venture into. Okay. Maybe he brushed his teeth with Simple Green. I did remember the original commercials for it including a shot of the inventor actually drinking the stuff, so that wouldn't be the end of the world. His Medi-Cal did not cover dental.

"God dammit, Nick, this is what I've been saying. You have to take care of your teeth. You only get the one set, and if you mess them up, you're screwed!" I threw all the dental care products into the air. They crashed to the floor. I wasn't feeling particularly Zen those days. "Fine. If you don't care enough to do something as basic as brushing your teeth, then don't come to me when the inevitable result rears its ugly head!" I stormed out, knowing I was about to pay for a bunch of dental work.

The next day he admitted that his teeth might be hurting just a little bit.

I took Nick to our family dentist, and we began a series of seemingly endless dental procedures. The dear man was trying to work with me to defray the costs of three root canals. He sent us to UCLA School of Dentistry, where they offered a reduced price. After weeks of paperwork and preparation, the day arrived. I lay all kinds of groundwork with the staff there, making sure they understood that Nick had schizophrenia. We drove to tony Westwood, paid the ridiculous parking fee, went inside, and waited for two hours. When they called Nick's name, he announced that he had changed his mind and then left.

I didn't even look for him. I stormed to the parking lot, slammed into my car, and began beating the steering wheel with my hands. Taking a deep breath, I placed my hands on the dashboard. The heat of my stinging palms cooled.

I had to stop on the way home to pick up something for a designer with whom I worked. It was on the south side of LA, the industrial area. On the way into the building, an older man stopped me.

"Excuse me, miss,"—miss, not ma'am? I was game—"could I trouble you for a cigarette?"

"Oh, you know, I'm sorry, man, I don't even smoke," I replied. Then it hit me. "Sir! Sir! Wait a minute!" I remembered that I had cartons of cigarettes in the trunk for dispensing to Nick.

I ran back to the truck and grabbed a carton, ready to rip it open. *Oh, what the hell*, I thought, and I took the whole thing. I was useless in the war against schizophrenia, but I *could* make this guy's day.

I scrambled over to him and, with a big stupid grin, said, "Here, take these."

"Oh, you are too kind," he said. "I will always remember your overwhelming kindness, lady."

"It is my pleasure, sir."

I felt better.

That night, my neighbor Theresa was having a gathering. We had all been friends for so long that no subject was taboo: divorces, unfaithful husbands, the goddamned kids, the scary, scary future. Things were still going strong when our friend Belinda asked me, in her proper British accent, "So, Mimi, what is going on with your Nick?" She said 'your Nick' because she also had a Nick, the same age as mine. They'd been friends, back before.

Well, I spilled it out, all over Theresa's beautiful party. The cockroaches. The dentists. The holes in the walls. The panic. The helplessness. The rage. It just kept coming and coming, and I couldn't censor it. People started leaving. Pretty soon, there was just Theresa, Belinda, and me in the kitchen.

"Wow, I really know how to clear a room."

"Yes, that was quite effective, Mimi," Theresa said, smiling.

"Oh, crap, I'm so sorry."

"I asked," Belinda offered.

"Yeah, it's your fault," I said. We started laughing.

"Yes, but you may have a new career on the horizon. The Party Clearer. Any time people are overstaying their welcome, you will, for a small fee, come over and tell everyone how you are doing!"

Through my continued, concentrated practice of yoga and meditation, I was developing a new worldview—a more thoughtful way of navigating the minefield. I understood that surrender, something I'd always identified with weakness, was anything but. Surrender, or acceptance, took strength and wisdom. It was recognizing what was inevitable or out of one's control and moving around it or through it. Allowing it. I was also in the best shape of my life, doing surprising balance poses, handstands galore. I noticed a strange tingling in my fingers when I landed too hard but dismissed it as nothing to worry about.

The next time we attempted the dental procedure, there was no problem. Nick was suddenly the perfect patient. That was the thing—nothing was ever consistent. Nothing made sense. We started over every single day.

Nick and I plodded though seemingly endless dental work together. It cost a huge amount of money. Sometimes when I felt myself sinking, I remembered the cigarette guy, how easy it had been to make his day, and I pulled myself up. I was trying so hard.

At the end I gave Nick a lecture about the treacherous road ahead if he did not start on a regimen of dental hygiene. But what, really, was I going to do? Go to his house twice a day and make sure he brushed his teeth? I didn't have it in me.

Rose completed high school, and I sighed with relief. She had no interest in college. We decided to give her a few months to figure things out without any pressure.

Craig and I were not fighting anymore, but the distance between us had become immense. I could feel the drawing near of an empty nest, and with that, Craig's absence in my life announced itself. And it was not what I wanted. Lucy and Rose were both in Los Angeles and could tend to Nick, so Craig and I planned a road trip to the San Juan Islands. I wanted us to reconnect. I started taking better care of myself. I was eating better, drinking less wine, even went to the doctor for a checkup because my neck had been hurting. She did a bunch of tests and everything looked good. It was getting warmer outside, and my mood was improving.

Craig picked me up at Sea-Tac Airport with the truck all packed. We'd decided to drive up to Orcas Island and camp.

The weather was good for June, sunny and warm. By the time we were on the ferry, it was midafternoon. I felt carefree in a way I hadn't been in a long time. Nick was safe under the girls' supervision; they would go over every day, give him his meds, take him for fast food. And I was on the water. We found a secluded campsite right on the beach. It was early season, so few people were around.

"Let's take a drive around the island," Craig suggested. "I hear there's an old tower with quite a view."

"I'm game for anything," I said, and meant it.

We made our way to Mount Constitution, the highest point in the San Juan Islands. There was a stone observation tower built by the WPA, patterned in the medieval style.

The 360-degree view was breathtaking. We walked all around to take it in.

"Had enough?" Craig asked.

"Yeah, I'm getting hungry. Let's go."

As we reached the first little landing, my phone, buried in my purse, rang. I fumbled around and found it.

"Hello, Miss Feldman, this is Dr. Mogannum." I leaned into the corner of the parapet to get out of the way. Craig was still on the level above, looking down at me. I stood with the phone in one hand and my finger in the other ear.

"Miss Feldman, I've just received the results of the MRI we took of your neck and head," she said. I had forgotten she'd ordered the test at my physical because of the neck pain. "They are very concerning," she informed me. I felt the color drain out of my face. I definitely saw it drain out of Craig's as he watched.

She explained that I had a serious cervical stenosis and would need surgery as soon as possible. The vertebrae in my neck had closed in to such a degree that they were resting directly on my spinal cord. Any fall could potentially cause quadriplegia. She said I had to be extremely careful. The image of me that very morning, getting tangled in the blankets while going for the alarm and falling, smashing my head into the dresser, came to mind. She went on in excruciating detail as the sightseers filed past me. Craig and I stood like sentries, unmoving, staring at each other. He knew that whatever this was, it was bad.

"Do you have any questions?"

Oddly, I didn't.

"All right, then, there's one more thing," she continued. *One more thing?*

"The MRI also showed something that had been noted three years ago when you had a head scan in the ER, after a car accident? There was some sort of mass. It has grown, and we can now see it's what looks like a meningioma, a type of brain tumor. They are almost always benign."

Wait a minute. Wait a minute here. Was she telling me I had a critical, dangerous neck condition that required major surgery AND A SIDE ORDER OF BRAIN TUMOR?

"The meningioma is not something that we have to act on right away. Since you are on vacation, I'd suggest that you finish your time there, try and enjoy yourself"—really?—"and call me when you return. I will—"

The phone went dead.

By now Craig had descended the stairs. He stood next to me. I sunk down into my favorite crouch position and put my tumor-ridden head in my hands.

"What?" Craig said. I rose and motioned for him to follow me down. "No. You can't do that. I need to know now."

Standing, crunched into a corner out of consideration to others, I told him. We hugged, said nothing, then went down the many stairs.

Sitting on a bench, he patted my back like you do a baby, saying "It's all right" over and over. Leaning against him, I felt nothing.

After a bit, he went to the bathroom, and I wandered around in a daze.

I guess I should cry, I thought. *I cry at the drop of a hat. Why aren't I crying now?* I cried a bit, but my heart wasn't in it, so I stopped. Hallmark commercial? Bring on the Kleenex. Life-threatening medical condition? Evidently not cry-worthy. I will never understand human emotional wiring. I think we are *all* nuts. I went into the gift shop and bought a glass that said "Mount Constitution" on it in fake gold leaf.

When Craig came out of the bathroom, I said, "She told me to avoid falling and hitting my head."

"Has she met you?" he asked.

"I know, right?"

We went back to our idyllic campsite, only now it didn't seem so great. When you get news like this, terrifying explorations on the internet are called for immediately. What good is this if I can't intensify it with all the appalling possibilities that will scare me to death? If not that, then at least copious amounts of alcohol and television to distract me, please. Nope. What I got was the tranquil, repetitive swish of the lagoon water and a spectacular sunset. All served up just for me to sit and contemplate my own death. With my big, silent, terrified husband in the too-small camping chair next to me. Once it was dark, there were only my thoughts and the ocean's splash, which had begun to feel like some sort of water torture.

Bone against spine, I walked to my sleeping bag.

The next morning, we solemnly packed up camp. So much for reconnecting. As we left, Craig, who is the most careful driver I know, backed right into a retaining wall with some serious force. We both whiplashed forward and back. We looked at each other, mouths open. I checked to see that I hadn't just been paralyzed. Once we established that I could move, Craig got out to assess the damage. I could see him, in the rearview mirror, crouching down to look at the bumper.

"Well, there ya go," I said to the empty truck.

For years, I had scrambled for some absolute, but everything kept unraveling. Lately it felt like I had finally found some stability, but now it was gone. As Craig crawled around inspecting the damage to the truck, I had such a need for certainty, it was like hunger.

Mindlessly I picked up the souvenir glass from the seat where I'd left it the day before. I hung my right arm out the window, clutching it. I looked down at the asphalt, then at the small circle of my face in the side-view mirror. Deliberately and with grace, I opened my fingers from around the glass. It fell into the morning, and a symphony rose as it broke into tiny pieces.

The certainty of glass to pavement.

12

THE PROJECT

Back home in LA two days later, I was ready. Unlike schizophrenia, this was understandable. There were facts leading to answers out there, and I was going to find them. Dr. Mogannum gave me the overview. First priority was the neck, because of the threat of paralysis. They wouldn't be able to do the surgery to remove the meningioma pressing on my brain until my neck was stable because it required intubation. The meningioma was most likely benign and very slow growing, so there was no rush. The task at hand was to find a neck surgeon.

"I'll just have to have these things taken care of, and then it will be business as usual. It is NOT cancer," I told the girls. "I'm not dying." I was so definite they seemed convinced. I was fine. This was different from Nick. It was *me*. Me I could handle.

The thing is, the damn yoga had become important to me. It was more than just exercise. It had snuck in the back door and become a way of life. The conventional approach to my condition was to just fuse all the vertebrae, but that would severely limit my yoga practice.

My friend Leigh Hamilton, who owned the gallery that showed my work, had had a meningioma three years earlier, so she coached me up.

"You cannot go alone to the doctors' appointments," she instructed. "And don't bring Craig. It's only going to scare him. You need someone methodical and calm. Someone to take notes so you can concentrate on talking to the doctors."

I needed a wingman. The obvious choice: my sister, Sara. Leigh was right; Craig was too emotional. He was being very attentive and loving, but I doubt that he could have written a coherent sentence at the time. In personal interaction and relationships, no one would accuse my sister of being methodical and calm. But when it came to anything else, she was whip-smart and capable. We've had a rocky relationship, but when the rubber meets the road, she's never let me down. I asked her to be my brain tumor/messed-up-neck buddy, and she said yes.

I hadn't told Nick yet. I was pretty sure he wouldn't freak out; nothing that happened to anyone else seemed to affect him much. With that in mind, I decided I'd fill him in the next time we went out to eat together.

I realized that I was nervous when we got to the restaurant. He was withdrawn. I tried to draw him out, but all he would do was nod.

"Nick, we're sitting here at lunch. You could have the good manners to converse with me." I waited.

He reached way, way down inside himself. It was excruciating to watch.

"Nice weather we've been having, don't you think?" he said slowly. I wanted to weep with gratitude.

"So, Nick, actually, I wanted to tell you about something that's been going on," I said. "It turns out I am going to have to get some surgery. My neck is out of whack, and they want to fix that first. Then it seems I have a small brain tumor. They're going to have to remove that afterward. But don't worry. It's not cancer."

"Hmmm," he said, nodding his head.

"Do you understand what I'm telling you, Nick?"

"Yes. But you're going to be fine, right?"

"Yes, I am."

He went back to his meal.

"Yeah, it's really weird how this all happened. Really, really weird." Oh, no. I was starting to babble. "Yeah, I went to the doctor because there was this bizarre thing that was happening. Every time I jumped off the truck or sat down on a chair hard, I'd have this crazy vibrating feeling out of my hands. Like from my fingertips. It was like electricity was shooting out of them—like a superhero or something. It was nuts!"

He looked up. "Oh, *that*," he said dismissively. "*That* happens to everyone."

I shut up and ate Brazilian spit-fired meat until *I* was in a food coma.

Leigh owned the gallery where I showed my work. She was a force of nature—a tall, statuesque knockout of a blonde, loud, opinionated, and funny. Everyone adored her. When I got my diagnosis, I discovered another side of Leigh. Once we crossed over into friendship, I found a woman full of love and compassion.

Leigh's meningioma had been in the back of her head, near the vision center. It required a difficult surgery because it was permeating the whole area. I remembered her visiting my studio for an upcoming show.

"Mimi, these colors are dull, too muted. You must punch them up, make it more alive!"

Oh, how we love our gallerists telling us how to paint. I was annoyed. Later, we realized it was the tumor—*she wasn't seeing color*. After it was removed, she said it was like the moment in *The Wizard of Oz* where it goes from black and white to Technicolor.

"Mimi, can you tone this down a bit? It looks gaudy."

My tumor was a piece of cake compared to Leigh's. It was right above my left brow and not near anything important. She charted out my course, told me who to talk to, where to go, what to ask. I was on double duty with this, investigating the treatment for my neck *and* my head. But thanks to the wonderful Leigh Hamilton, *this* time I had the motherfucking map.

It was early summer. Sara met me at every appointment, with her BlackBerry. She'd take copious notes on the device and then transcribe them onto a yellow steno pad for me. I think we were every doctor's worst nightmare: two smart, unrelenting, loud broads with endless questions. I'd talk to the physician, and Sara would sit, furiously taking notes. Then she'd step in with her list, ready for round two. The idea was to see at least three doctors for each issue and then compare recommendations.

After several meetings about my neck, we'd gotten nowhere. The opinions varied, but they all said I needed a laminectomy, the fusing of the vertebrae, which I was trying to avoid. More than once, I was told, "If I wasn't sure these MRIs belonged to the person in front of me, I'd say a mistake had been made."

It appeared that my muscles had strengthened and modified themselves to support my crumbling neck. They were actually compensating for the lack of bone support. This fueled my resolve for finding an alternative to turning my neck into a steel rod.

We were in a consultation with one spinal specialist who suddenly held his palm up and then flew out the door.

"What was that?" Sara said.

"I know, huh? That was weird. He probably decided I was hopeless."

"Hey, Mimi," Sara said.

"What?"

"Your shirt is on inside out." She started laughing wickedly.

"Oh God, just take me to the Alzheimer's ward."

Ten minutes later, the door opened and the doctor returned, flanked by a tall, striking man wearing a Sikh's turban. Dr. Harsimran Singh Brara. Dr. Brara wore a crisp light-blue shirt and a silk tie—a very elegant man. He had been working on an alternative procedure that was perfect for me. Rather than fusing everything together, he proposed opening the vertebrae one by one to create space for my spinal cord, putting little spacers in to hold them open. Eventually they would attach to my bones and become permanent. The spacers would be made of cadaver bones that had been baked in an oven at high heat to eliminate any DNA, thus making them acceptable to another body. He was confident that it would leave me with almost complete mobility in my neck.

"Would this be something you are interested in, Ms. Feldman?" he asked in his lilting Indian accent.

"Can you do it today?" I asked.

Sara and I were elated as we drove home. We both immediately trusted Dr. Brara and had no doubts whatsoever. Our quest was over.

"Ooo, and I'm going to have dead people's bones in me. That's so cool."

"You are a child," Sara said.

A few days later, we found ourselves waiting in the office of Dr. Schweitzer, neurosurgeon. Sara was making derisive comments about the receptionist, and I was rifling through my now enormous file of medical information. It was brain tumor time. On the wall was his medical degree from Stanford. I pointed to it and raised my eyebrows, and Sara nodded. In walked a very good-looking, middle-aged guy wearing Sperry Top-Siders. By then, I had seen two other surgeons about the tumor, and they both had the same opinion. At that point, if Dr. Schweitzer concurred, I'd go with him because I had Kaiser coverage.

"You have two options as to the method of surgery here, Ms. Feldman. Your decision will be predicated on your priorities. There are many women who would be averse to having a scar on their face. For them, the best option is this—we make an incision just behind your hairline above your forehead. We then peel the skin of the face back to access the tumor and remove it. Then, the face is pulled back into place and stitched behind the hairline. When healed, no scar would be visible."

"Could you pull that face up just a little tighter for her?" Sara asked.

I have to admit I was thinking the same thing. The doctor smiled uncomfortably and continued.

"The second approach is what we call keyhole surgery. With this method, we cut through the forehead and drill a hole into the skull to access the meningioma. It is easier and holds less risk, but it will leave you with a scar on your forehead," he said.

"So my dream of being a supermodel will be over?" I asked.

Sara snorted, and he stared at the wall above my head.

"Okay. If the two choices are peeling my whole face off or ending up with a scar, I'm going keyhole, for sure." It was getting way too uncomfortable in the room.

The bigger question was shaping up to be the timing. I had to have the neck surgery before I did something stupid to myself and became wheelchair-bound, but there was also a case to be made for not even doing the brain surgery. I could wait indefinitely. I interrogated him about the pros and cons of that. The idea of just leaving this thing to grow in my head seemed irrational to me.

"Doctor, if it was your wife, what would you advise her to do?"

"Look," he said, "you are in very good health right now."

Other than the toothpick neck and the brain tumor? I thought. I looked over to Sara and knew from her smirk she was thinking the same thing.

"You could leave the meningioma," he continued, "and perhaps live the rest of your life with it. But there is just enough activity to indicate continued growth. In a few years, you might not be in as good health. If it was my wife, I would take it out now."

I thanked him for his time. Sara and I walked down the hallway. My head was spinning.

Inside the crowded elevator, my sister turned to me and said loudly, "Okay. Jewish. Handsome. Stanford. That's the trifecta, Mimi. You gotta go with this guy."

And so I did. I decided to just get it all over with. I didn't want to live with this any longer than I had to. If I scheduled the neck surgery in early September, factoring in recovery time, I could still have the brain surgery in the same calendar year and avoid having to meet my deductible again the next year.

Through all of this, Craig was by my side. He never weighed in, opinion-wise. He understood that this was my body and I was going to make the decisions. The idea of losing me, being left alone with the mess that was our life, must have been paralyzing. Yet he managed to do the exact, best thing. He was next to me as I found my way through, marshaled by my sister, without whom I would have been completely lost.

Meanwhile, Rose was lounging around the house, comfortable in her lassitude. She hadn't gotten a job or made any plans. She continued to control the kitchen, one box of cow entrails after the other. Lucy came and went, working, having a social life. I lost track of the last time I'd sent the cleaning crew to Nick's.

It was August. Craig and I had made plans to go to the beach for a few days. After conferring with the doctors, we decided that the trip was feasible. I had to promise to be very careful—no swimming in the ocean—and we would schedule the surgery for September.

I was so happy to leave all the medical crap behind. The day was perfect, with bright, clear sunlight and a cobalt ocean. I lay on the sand next to Craig. The cartoon devil and angel sat on my shoulders.

"Go in," the devil said. "This could be your last chance."

"Are you nuts?" the angel chirped. "You could end up paralyzed!"

"Look at that blue, blue sea," the devil pointed out. "How can you pass it up?"

I stood up.

"Hey," Craig called after me as I ran and dove, the cool, cleansing Pacific rushing over my head. I was twelve years old again, body surfing with my brother. I was a wild human fish breaking all rules. I was a mermaid poet, verse thrumming in my ears like water. Clickings of rock against shell, recalled from the depth of seas, were the drumbeat. I moved under the weight of waves.

When I emerged, Craig was at the shore. "Are you insane?" he asked. I was panting, smiling.

"Nope. Fuck it, I'm here, and I'll be good-goddamned if I don't go into the ocean. Hell, I might die on the operating table."

"That's the spirit," Craig said with his trademark sarcasm.

That time in the ocean was mine alone.

Lying in bed the last night of our trip, looking at our computers, we prepared ourselves to go home and face the future. I got an email from Brooke. "I don't know any good way to tell you this, but Leigh has been diagnosed with cancer. It is bad, and I will call as soon as I know more."

I burst into tears.

"What?" Craig asked, scared.

I handed him my computer.

"Oh no," he said.

After an exhausting summer of research, I was finally ready to take on my surgeries, but this news made everything swerve. I shut my computer and stared at the ceiling.

13

RUNNING THROUGH FIRE

It was the night before my neck surgery. I'd tried to settle any fears the girls had with a definite "everything is going to be fine." "I love you" chorused through the hall between our bedrooms. Scarlett called and told me she was sure everything would be fine. I called Nick. He was just dandy about all this, because I'd told him there was nothing to worry about, and he believed me. He was more concerned about whether I left all the things he needed with the girls.

Craig and I watched some TV and went to bed. There was surprisingly little to say. It was autumn and cooler outside. I could see through the sheer curtains and into the night, sparse clouds lit white by the moon's glow. Leaves on the trees bridled against sudden breezes. The very last flowers of summer adorned the lawns. Everyone was tucked in for the night. In front of my house, a few small pieces of broken glass lay on the asphalt. They sparkled to trick the eye and be called diamonds. They sparkled and shined and maybe flew up to the moon in the middle of the night.

Craig wrapped himself around me like a child yearning for home.

Morning arrived, and I thought, *This might be my last one.* Our house still had its hundred-year-old windows, with the wavy sort of glass that distorts things just enough to make them look soft and lovely. The view through that glass was rosy, but I looked away.

We didn't talk in the car. Out the window, the blue light reminded me of that early morning I'd driven madly to Venice to find Nick with his wrist slashed. It felt like a million years ago. For some reason I remembered the white teddy bear that was Nick's companion when he was a toddler.

"What are you going to name him, Nick?" I'd asked him.

"One Guy"

"Really? Why?"

"Because that's what he is—one guy."

When we arrived, it was light. Walking toward the building, Craig reached for my hand. Our hands do not fit together well, so we are not one of those couples who walk around with fingers intertwined. But that day our mismatched knuckles held us both up. As we crossed Sunset Boulevard, I saw Dr. Brara. He cut a fine figure in his tailored suit. His shirt that day was pink. He saw us and smiled.

"See you inside," I said, suddenly feeling better.

Sara was going to meet Craig and wait with him. I had been adamant about the kids not being there during the operation. They didn't need that trauma.

We did the intake procedures. Craig came in and sat with me for a while as the IVs were hooked up and my body's status measured and assessed. A nurse gently swept my hair into a surgical cap. She attached a couple of monitors to my chest. A dull buzzing sound from an unclear source filled the room, and the florescent lights occasionally burst bright. Each time they did, I grabbed a fast breath. When it came time for Craig to leave, he leaned over and kissed me. "It's going to be fine, Feldman. I love you." His dark eyes held fear, but the timbre of his voice was only love.

Waking up was a shock. I hadn't been prepared for how unbelievably bad I'd feel. I had a big, cumbersome neck brace on over the massive bandages. According to Craig, I was drooling and talking incoherently.

One eye was half shut, and the other glared wildly. Every single thing about my body, mind, and soul was off-kilter.

The next time I awoke was in the hospital room the following day. My mouth was dry, and the neck brace had me in its unforgiving grip. Craig was sitting in the chair next to me, reading the newspaper. For the next day or so I was in a delirium, all drugged up. I don't even remember the kids visiting. All I recall is one unfortunate trip to the bathroom, and seeing Craig, sitting there like Atticus Finch every time I woke up.

After four days, they gave me directions on how to deal with the neck brace—my new nemesis—and sent me home. I was to wear it at all times, even in the bath. The nurse wheeled me out to meet Craig at the curb. He brought me home, I stumbled into bed, and there I stayed. Evidently my "couple of days later" scenario had been fantastical. I didn't want to see anyone or do anything. Eating was not appealing to me at all. Rose's chicken feet bone broth finally had its day; that was all I could stomach.

She'd bring me a big bowl of it every night, her face glowing with sweet vindication.

After about a week, I started to feel like joining the ranks of the living. Everyone agreed that the first order of business was a bath. I wasn't allowed to shower, so Craig and Rose were tasked with bathing me. I stood naked in front of them, and they helped me into the tub. The room was steamy with oils and balms. I remember feeling weak and vulnerable, but it didn't bother me the way I would have thought. They washed my hair and bathed me, and I was happy to surrender. Rose combed my hair.

I decided it was time to go outside. They told me taking short walks would be beneficial. It took twenty minutes for me to navigate the stairway. After that, Craig helped me down the front porch steps, where I sat for a while. I declared my readiness, and off we hobbled. Finding myself taking unsteady baby steps while hanging on his arm was a humbling experience. We walked down Norton Avenue, tiny step by tiny step. We passed a neighbor who said hello, eyes shining with alarm. Oh well, no time for explanations. I had an excruciatingly slow walk to take.

I returned to the hospital for my first postsurgical visit. They removed the big bandage and replaced it with a smaller one. I had to wear the neck brace for seven more weeks. It was torture. I wanted to throw that damn thing into outer space. I started secretly taking it off when no one was there.

I quickly returned to my old, energetic self. I had a couple of jobs going, and Craig drove me over to supervise. My guys looked at me like I was nuts, walking the construction site with a neck brace. Rose was still struggling with depression, now seeing a therapist and continuing to work the Gut Diet. Nick would show up for dinner and do his Boo Radley thing on the porch. Lucy came and went, always a smile on her face.

I hadn't picked up a paintbrush in weeks.

One evening, a few weeks in, I went down to the kitchen to make some tea. I boiled the water, preparing to put it in a big jar to cool. The neck brace was working my last nerve. Craig wasn't home and Rose was upstairs, so I took it off.

"Mom! What the heck? Where is your neck brace?" She stood at the bottom of the steps.

Shit. Busted. "It's not a big deal, Rose. I just took it off for a minute. I'm being very careful."

"Are you kidding me? You're not supposed to take it off at all. Let me do that. You go put it back on. Right now!" There was no arguing with that. I handed her the teakettle and went over to the table where the brace lay like roadkill.

As I was strapping it back on, Rose screamed. I looked up and saw the big glass jar shattering as she poured hot water in. It splashed all down her leg.

Then we were both screaming.

"Quick, we have to get cold water on it," I shouted.

"Ow, ow, ow, ow," she shrieked.

I ripped her pants down to get the hot water away and went to the sink for some cold.

"Lie down," I said. "Let me just put some cold towels on it."

Eventually we ended up in the kids' bathroom, trying to assess the damage.

"Rose, this is seriously red. We need to go to the emergency room."

"No. I don't want that. Every time I go to the hospital, they do something terrible to me."

Perhaps it was postsurgical delirium, but somehow I agreed. Rose and I embarked on yet another injury-based adventure, this one caused by my decision to take off my neck brace.

The next day the burn was even redder and had spread. Soon it became a thigh-sized, watery blister. She kept it scrupulously clean and treated it with colloidal silver, something I had never even heard of.

"Rose. We HAVE to go to the doctor," I insisted. I cannot remember where Craig was in all of this. The memory is of a world inhabited by only Rose and me.

"No. I'm going to do this the homeopathic way. Hand me the colloidal silver."

The days went by. The blister took on a life of its own, and we were just spectators. Rose lay on her bed and waited. Somehow, miraculously, it disappeared as her body reabsorbed the liquid. I couldn't believe it.

In those days Rose and I were at odds in so many ways but close in a manner I hadn't been with any of the other children. We were opposites caught in a never-ending dance, destined to irritate yet save each other. It was beautiful.

Once the neck brace was off, she began to pull away again. The spell had been broken.

I had a few weeks to live like a regular person before the brain surgery. I still hadn't gone back into my studio. I felt detached from that part of me, and I didn't care.

It was time to check on Nick's apartment. It had been months.

"I'd like to get a new bed, Ma. The one I have is so old. Do you think I could get a new bed?"

"Well, I haven't seen your apartment in quite a while. Have you been keeping it clean?" I asked.

"Yeah, it's fine," he replied.

"Really? Fine?"

"It's clean, Mom. Everything is good."

"Well, this is not my first rodeo, Bub, so I'm going to have to come down there and see for myself. If it's clean, then we can talk about the bed."

As usual, he hung up without a goodbye. When he left in person, he'd always say goodbye, but when he was finished on the phone he just hung up.

The apartment was (surprise!) a disaster. After some steely admonishment, we straightened up for the cleaning crew. The maids came the next day. When I drove down to pay them, the head guy took me aside and said, "Lady, we cleaned everything up, but I think you need to check his box spring. There are roaches in there." Great.

I informed Nick that we would be replacing only his box spring, and if he kept his apartment clean we'd replace the mattress in a few weeks.

"But, Mom, as long as we are getting the box spring, couldn't we just get me a mattress too?"

"No, Nick, we could not."

"I really wanted to get a new mattress," he said sadly.

"Yeah, well, I really wanted to be a famous artist. So cry me a river."

Delivery was set for the next day. They offered the service of removing the old box spring, but I knew better than that. I was sure that once a gazillion roaches started swarming out of the thing into their truck, we'd have a problem.

The next morning, I drove down to Nick's apartment.

"Nick, we have to get this out of here before they come," I declared.

I was still supposed to be taking it easy, so I had him pull the mattress off the box spring.

"Okay, so now lift it up," I said foolishly.

They were crawling in actual clumps all around the metal springs. The guts of the box spring stood splayed open before me like a black-and-silver living creature.

"All right, man, we have got to get this thing out of here. Pronto," I commanded. "You take the front, I'll take the back. Go!"

We dragged that baby, spewing vermin, through the lobby and out onto the street. Me and my crazy son.

"Here, Nick. We gotta put it across the street. We don't want them to know it's yours."

I had long since abandoned all hope of good citizenship. I lived in survival mode. We tossed it in front of the church across the street.

We returned to his apartment, and I sprayed a bunch of cans of insecticide. After scooping up bugs in the dustpan, I sent Nick to the dumpster with the last bag just as the mattress guys arrived. Ignoring the unbreathable residue of chemicals in the air, I said, "Oh, hello, gentleman. The box spring goes right over here."

It was two weeks before my brain surgery. I was losing it. Now that I had experience with major surgery, I was scared to death. The bravery with which I had told the girls everything was going to be fine and marched into neck surgery was a distant memory. I hadn't been courageous—I had simply been clueless. I *really* didn't want to do it again. I wasn't even looking forward to the drugs.

"Are you ready for this?" Craig asked me.

"I just want to get it over with," I replied.

"You know, Meem, you don't have to do this right now. You could wait. It's not too late to change your mind."

"No. I'm so sick of this shit. I want it behind me."

I had returned to yoga classes. The first day I showed up, I was ready to wow everyone. We started on the floor, in child's pose, worked our way up to standing, and then began sun salutations. Feeling good, my arms up to the sky, folding forward, it felt like nothing had changed. Palms flat, jump back to chaturanga. I collapsed to the floor. There was no way I could hold the pose; my arms couldn't support my body. As I lay facedown on the floor, I started to tear up. This wasn't the way it was supposed to go. I stumbled my way through the class.

Afterward I went to my teacher.

"Oh no," I said, trying not to let the floodgates open. "I've lost everything."

"You haven't lost *anything*," she said. "You've been through a serious trauma to your body. In my experience, it takes three months to regain your previous strength. Just show up, every day, to your mat, and all will be revealed."

There was a time in my life when I would have laughed scornfully at those words. They would have meant nothing to me. One either succeeded or failed. But that day, when I fell to the floor because my own arms couldn't sustain me, when all ego and sense of accomplishment was lost, that is the day I mark as the real start of my yoga practice. And it was a good day.

Over the years since Nick had become ill, I'd developed a checkered relationship with the LAPD. On the one hand, they were my saviors, coming at short notice to help us. On the other, I seemed to be having an increase in the frequency of my traffic stops. It began with a photographic citation arriving in the mail with an image of me running a red light, with my cell phone in one hand and a large turkey sandwich in the other. It would be hard to dispute that one.

But I had developed a new philosophy in reaction to the lousy cards I'd been dealt regarding Nick: I allowed myself to play the "crazy card."

I could use it to get out of social events, work, anything I didn't want to do. Disgraceful, I know, but my reasoning was that if I had to deal with schizophrenia on a daily basis, then this was my consolation prize. I showed up at Beverly Hills Courthouse with Nick's SSI papers (certification of his crazy), some hospital intake forms (dates slightly altered), and a detailed story of having to run the light due to Nick's imminent hospitalization. Of course, I was the last person called. I sat and waited through all the other ridiculous excuses, the dumbfounded plaintiffs, the irritated judge, until finally I heard my name.

"Your Honor, I am not denying that I ran the red light, but there were extenuating circumstances that I believe will justify my action. You see, my twenty-six-year-old son has schizophrenia . . ."

"Oh, you have my sympathies," she said. "I have a close friend in the same situation."

Bingo.

Once, after a particularly trying day with Nick, I saw the now-familiar flashing red lights behind me. I was near a school, so this was bad. Stricter rules applied. I looked in the rearview mirror and saw a tough-looking policewoman sauntering up. I knew I'd never win. I rolled down my window, ready to take what was coming.

"Good afternoon, ma'am," she said.

I started crying. It wasn't a ploy. I just started blubbering and rambling incoherently about Nick. I couldn't stop.

"You just drive home carefully and try and calm down, dear, okay?"

It didn't always go that well. I'd accumulated several moving violations and had a real shell game going. Traffic school is allowed only once in eighteen months. I was taking online school repeatedly, trying to parlay my tickets by requesting extensions and appearing in front of judges. I discovered that wearing my neck brace, even after I no longer had to, helped a lot in the sympathy department. If I brought my dead mother's cane along, they let me go to the front of the line.

I offer no excuse for my behavior—it was dreadful. Finally, like any nincompoop's folly, it all came crashing down. One particularly disdainful judge required me to attend a two-day, in-person driving school before the end of November. The only available one was the weekend before my brain surgery. I also had one last ticket I'd somehow deferred for two years. I'd deal with that afterward, assuming I lived.

I headed off to the Comedy Traffic School in a run-down industrial part of West LA. Nothing funny going on there. The room was filled with losers and misfits, just like me. In order to be sent to the two-day live school, you had to screw up big.

In front of me sat Biker Guy, on my right was Smelly Shirt Man, and behind me Goth Girl repeatedly tapped my chair with her foot. I didn't dare say a word. The teacher was a middle-aged guy in Dockers and a striped long-sleeved T-shirt. His name was Barry.

"I know you all are expecting this to be a fun comedic class, but I'm sorry to report that the usual teacher is out sick, so they had to send me over from the regular traffic school," he announced sheepishly.

"So, what, you're not even funny?" Goth Girl asked.

"Well, my wife doesn't think so, but I can try," Barry replied.

A guy with a braided beard threw himself into the chair to my left.

If I die and this is how I spent my last weekend on earth, I'm going to be really pissed, I thought to myself.

14

A BOOT-SHAPED HEART

When Rose was about two weeks old, she got a cold. It was nothing, really, but because she was so young, I took her to the doctor. He confirmed that the cold was not serious and asked what we planned to do about the heart murmur.

"Heart murmur?"

"Yes. She has one. Your pediatrician didn't tell you? We're running some tests."

The x-ray showed that she might have what is called a "boot-shaped heart," which is very serious and can be fatal. That, or she might have simply moved during the x-ray. Quite a gamut to consider while they did more tests. They took her away for an MRI.

Craig and I sat in the waiting room for a long time, his foot gently rocking the empty baby seat.

"You know when you see a whole bunch of birds swooshing around the sky in a pattern?" I asked him.

"Yeah . . ."

"Did you know that's called a murmuration?"

"Good to know."

We returned to silence modulated by the faint squeak of the baby seat.

The MRI showed that she was fine. No boot-shaped heart. Just a little whisper as the blood moved through the left atrium to the right atrium. A murmur of the heart can heal itself in the first few years of life, and Rose's strong, resilient heart did just that.

Rose started therapy the day before my operation. That evening, I was sending an email, thanking her doctor.

"Who are you writing to?" Rose demanded at my office door.

"Not that it is your business, but I was just thanking your therapist."

"Really? What did you say?"

"Exactly what I just told you, Rose."

"I don't believe you. What did she say?" Her voice was going up. "LET ME SEE."

"You may not go on my computer, Rose. Now please go out of here," I replied.

"Let me see what she said." She was shouting now.

She tried to push me aside to see the computer. I pushed back. Craig walked into the room just as she knocked me off my chair.

"What are you doing, Rose? Your mother just had surgery!" He helped me up and turned to her. "This is the final straw. You need to leave. You can't stay here anymore."

I looked at him, looked at her, then sat down and put my head on the desk like we used to do in grammar school. *I got nothing*, I thought. *I have absolutely nothing left.* I sat and listened to the devastating fight like it was in another language.

The last thing I heard Craig say was "And take that dog of yours with you." The front door slammed, he stomped up the stairs, and then the bedroom door slammed. I pressed my cheek to the wood. I just had to get through the night.

Lucy called. "Mom, don't you know what happened? Dad threw Rose out! She's wandering around downtown with Woody. Buster got out and ran away."

"I know," I said flatly.

"Don't you care? What's wrong with you?" she beseeched me.

I went into the bedroom to find Craig sitting in the dark, holding his head. This was what he did in moments of terrible remorse. I got into bed and turned toward the wall, my back to the door that led to the hall through which Rose had left me.

I heard a lot of rumblings that night. Lucy entering. Hushed voices. Crying. Gates opening and closing. I lay in bed, pretending to sleep, and waited for daylight to arrive.

The next morning, Craig and I sat silently in the kitchen. A neighbor called to say she had found Buster. I put on some clothes and walked over there. It was a big white house with impeccable landscaping, overflowing flowerbeds in fantasy colors. A youngish dad opened the door to the comfortable, stylish home. They had a big, happy somethingdoodle, who smelled like shampoo and jumped all over the furniture. Buster was in the yard—old, black, and stinky. The pretty wife and smiley kids took me out to see him.

"Oh, we are just so glad we found him!" she chirped. "I shudder to think what might have happened to him, out all night alone."

The fact that I had been in my warm bed the previous night while my daughter wandered the streets felt like a hideous rash under my clothes only I knew was there.

"He's just a sweetie pie, he is," she said, gingerly petting him and further inflaming my guilt.

"Oh, thank you very much," I said. "I didn't sleep a wink last night." Not a lie.

I walked the block home holding his collar, stooped over like a banana-backed old grandma. A torrent of fear and regret rushed over me. That cheery house and the young family had made me feel weathered, soiled.

Then: numbness.

Suddenly Lucy's reproaches couldn't touch me. My terror about Rose's safety rested behind an imaginary wall. I didn't even call Nick before the surgery. I spoke to Craig only in monosyllables. Lying on my daybed with headphones, I listened to the Jim Carroll Band pound out *People Who Died* over and over. I have jumped and hollered to that song for years, as though somehow screaming at death could match its power, a furious, uncontrollable smashup of pain and joy. That morning I lay still but for my index finger, tapping intently to the drumbeat.

My entire life was a tenuous scab that couldn't be touched lest the hemorrhage commence.

Very little remains in my memory of the time between picking up Buster and coming to in the recovery room. It is an ashen void.

The world was dark, then reddish. I was vaguely aware of the fact that light was causing this transition. Red turned to pink, and I opened my eyes. I saw a blurry version of Craig and Sara.

"I didn't die," I slurred.

They both smiled.

"No, I mean I made it. I didn't die." I grinned like a chimp. "I didn't die?"

Sara squinted. Craig was pale.

"Oh, man, I love you guys. No. I mean I really love you. I didn't die."

I went on and on. Their faces changed from relieved to concerned. I guess I was delirious. "I love you so much. I really do." I was like a drunk frat boy. Then it all went from pink, to red, to black.

I woke up in the middle of the night in my hospital bed. I was all alone and scared. I pushed the call button. Far off, way down the barely lit hallway, I could hear sounds. They were festive sounds—laughing, music, chatter.

I pushed the button over and over, but no one came. I was freezing. I must have been sweating first, because the sheets were drenched, but now I wanted blankets. I started shivering. I could hear a raucous party going on way down the hall. Why didn't anyone come help me?

"Hello, young lady, are you awake now?" the middle-aged Filipino man asked me. "I am your nurse, Efren."

"I'm cold."

A woman stood behind him, and they giggled. Another nurse peeked into the room and smiled. I was sure I smelled onion dip.

What is going on here? I thought. *Last time they took such good care of me.*

"Here you go, lady, we will put another blanket on you," the nurse said and then left. I lay there in wet sheets with an extra blanket on top to seal in the misery, thinking about all the burn marks on Nick's carpet and imagining fires. They never returned.

The next morning when Craig and Sara arrived, I recounted my tale of neglect. "They partied while I froze alone here all night." They exchanged knowing looks, smiled the smile you give the crazy person. To this day, Sara and Craig laugh about my delusional night. But I know it happened. Those goddamned nurses were having a party.

Lucy brought Nick to see me.

Rose never came.

Lucy sat down on the bed and began kissing my face. Nick hovered nearby.

"So, what have you been up to?" I asked him.

"I watched a documentary about Burning Man. It was nice. I'm going to go outside and have a cigarette, okay?" He left.

I looked at Lucy. "I'm afraid his whole life is Burning Man."

"Yeah. In his head." We smiled at each other.

I insisted on being moved to another wing of the hospital. I didn't want to risk a night like the previous one. I wanted nurturing, soft women nurses, who stroked my brow and kept the sheets dry.

"Hello. I am Igor. I will be your nurse tonight." Really? I had moved from carousing to communism? Where the hell was Nurse Sweetie Pie?

I opened my eyes to the sight of a large Eastern European man in green nurse's scrubs. He took hold of my blanket with one large paw, and in an instant my bed was stripped. He transferred me to the visitor's chair and remade the bed in the blink of an eye.

Okay, now this *is a hallucination,* I thought.

It wasn't. Igor was a real live nurse from the Ukraine. He had a sense of humor and was generous with the pain meds. I got as many blankets as I wanted, and there was no partying whatsoever. I shared my grandmother's chicken paprikash recipe with him, and he brought me a real hot dog from the cafeteria. He told me the saga of his childhood, and I told him what ungrateful shits my kids were. We laughed ironically at the inequity in the world. Igor ushered me out of brain limbo and back to the world of the living. It took three days.

Dr. Schweitzer waltzed in and out. By now, I knew the doctors weren't the frontline players. The nurses controlled the game. They healed you, calmed you, cured you. The doctor was just the mechanic. The last day I was there, Dr. Schweitzer came to uncover my incision.

"Look at that," he said. "It's beautiful." He held the mirror up for me to see. There was an arched line above my eyebrow that mimicked its curve. I had rather been hoping for a tough pirate sort of scar, one that said this woman has been through some shit.

"Oh. Why is it arched like that?" I asked.

"I did that on purpose!" he said smugly. "This way, when it heals, it will look like just another wrinkle."

Great. Just another wrinkle. Those I can make on my own. I was counting on the brain surgeon for miracles.

They didn't bandage my incision. I wanted a cartoon-worthy big white wrap of gauze around my head, one that would show the world how I'd suffered. What I got was some new clear gel stuff slathered on my forehead. When it dried, it served as a magnifying glass to a very gnarly looking wound. It was like the kid with the thick lenses that made his eyes eerily big. I was going to scare some babies with that thing.

They discharged me on a Monday afternoon. I said my goodbyes to Igor and the gang, and a nurse wheeled me to the curb to meet Craig. I folded out of the chair into the car. Craig signaled, carefully pulled out, drove exactly one block, and then stopped the car.

"What?" I said.

"I just want to tell you something," he said. "I want you to know I am proud of you. You have been so brave and so strong. You made it, Mimi, you made it!"

I just stared at him.

"I mean, I know I couldn't have done what you did. I'd still be shaking under the covers. But you faced all this and just took care of business. I am in awe."

Once home, all I could think about was Rose. I understood Craig's position. She had ignored our rules for living at home: getting a job or going to school. She had attacked me. It was the way it happened, in yet another outburst of confusion and rage, that was eating me up alive. All I wanted was for her to come back.

The following Sunday morning, I nestled deeper into bed, and Craig got up to go to the bathroom. He passed the bed and then, suddenly, he started to stagger and fall. What was happening here? At first, I thought he was goofing around, but as he dropped to the floor, knocking into the large flat-screen TV, I realized this wasn't a joke. For one wild, slow-motion second, I watched my husband tumbling, the treasured television teetering, and thought, awfully inappropriately, *Sophie's Choice! Who do I save?*

I jumped up and called out to Lucy, the only one left at home.

Craig was unconscious on the floor. The flat screen wobbled precariously above him.

"What is happening?" Lucy shrieked at the bedroom door.

"I don't know, he just fell over. I'm calling 911!"

At that, Craig came to consciousness.

"No!" he shouted. "I'm fine. Don't call anyone."

"You're not fine," I replied. "You passed out, and I'm calling the paramedics."

I wandered, dumbfounded, around the hospital ward. The usual question of what Craig would do without me was supplanted by its opposite, and I was reeling.

Craig had had an episode of heart arrhythmia. I told anyone who would listen how weird it was that I had just had brain surgery and now here I was again. My gel-encased bloodbath of a forehead made my point for me. Craig was stable, so I sent Lucy home. Enough for her, already. Tapping at the edge of my consciousness was the realization that Craig, quietly, was as important a pylon in this family structure as I was. What would I do without him?

Meanwhile, I began a concerted internet and telephone mission to find Rose and let her know what was going on. I was happy to have a reason to pull her in, even given the serious nature of that reason. I pined for her like a lovesick teenager.

I slept in a chair next to Craig's bed that night, Atticus Finch myself.

The next day the doctors informed me that Craig would be fine. He'd have to go on medication. Lucy brought Nick over to see him. Scarlett talked to him on the phone. I called Sara and Danny to tell them the new bad news. I'd gotten chillingly good at that task.

Later that evening I received a text from Rose. I jolted as I read that she was in the parking lot but didn't know what to do with her bike. I ran down there. As soon as I laid eyes on her, I wanted to gather her up in my arms and never let go, but I knew better. She was skittish.

"Here, just put the bike in the truck, and we can go up and see Dad." Walking behind her, I took in her sad gait, those hunched, bony shoulders.

Rose had an awkward, yet loving, visit with her father. I cowered in the corner, suddenly relegated to insignificance. Somehow the onus of responsibility for this whole mess had shifted to me.

I felt as though my weakening physical state had failed the entire family. If I had just remained steady and strong, things wouldn't have gone awry in this terrible way. Nick was crazy. Lucy was furiously treading water, holding up more than she ever should have been called to do. Rose moved from one place to another in the room, like a boxer, establishing her position.

Craig began to fade. Soon he slept. My daughter scowled at me from her bedside seat.

"I guess I'm going to go now," she said, the timbre of her voice wavering ever so slightly.

Go where? Do what? Who will take care of you? How will I find you? I can make soup! "Sure. I'll walk you down to get your bike."

In the artificial light of the garage, we walked. Her tawny skin called to me like cool water in a shaded forest. She was so solitary and guarded. I knew it would be a long time before I'd see her again. We took her bike out of the truck, and she gave a faint shrug. I grabbed her, held her limp, unresponsive body, and felt a ruin that was different from anything I'd ever known. I understood that I was letting her go, and as I watched her slowly pedal away, I felt bankrupt, deep into my soul. My mouth was open, but I didn't speak. I brought my hand up and could feel my own warm breath washing my palm.

15

INTRINSIC PARITY

Wrecked, Craig and I returned home from the hospital the next day. We got into bed.

I made Nick walk to the house for medication; the cigarettes and money were sufficient bait. I'd meet him at the door with a glass of water and his pills.

"Thanks, Ma. See you tomorrow."

Not a word from Rose.

All I wanted to do was check out. Whether that was delivered by medication, sleep, or television didn't matter.

Craig and I were both so miserable we rarely left the bedroom.

"I just remembered something from when I was in the hospital," Craig said as we lay splayed on the bed in front of the constant distraction of the flat screen.

"Yeah? What?"

"You know how they come in at night and wake you up just to check on you? Sometimes they ask questions to gauge your awareness?"

"All too well," I snorted.

"So. That first night I was there I had this strange, older male nurse. He had an accent, but I don't know what it was," he said. "His name was Juan."

"Then just do Spanish, because all your accents sound like that anyway." I grinned.

"Shut up. So, at three in the morning he woke me up. I opened my eyes, and he stooped over and asked, 'Mr. O'Rourke, what do you fear most?'"

"Great accent," I said.

"No, really, he asked me that. Isn't that weird?"

"It is. What did you answer?"

"My immediate response was '*death*.'"

"Good choice. Not too creative, but solid," I said.

"I thought so."

"We're a pair, aren't we, O'Rourke?"

"That we are, Feldy."

We returned to entertainment oblivion.

As the days passed, we weaned ourselves from the TV and resumed our lives. I returned to work with my scary forehead. I walked indifferently past my studio each day.

I kept track of Rose through Lucy. Rose was couch surfing downtown. I enlisted Sara to take me to look for her. I knew I couldn't do it alone. I was quite sure she was staying with her old boyfriend in a bunker-style building on the edge of Chinatown. On the drive, I caught Sara up on what was going on. She started crying.

"Oh, there!" I said. "I think that's the place I dropped her off once." She pulled over.

We got out of the car just as the large metal front door opened.

"Shh. Wait," I said. "I don't want her to see me."

A young man dressed in a harlequin costume led the ragtag group. Behind him emerged two girls, arm in arm, eyes smudged black with makeup. Rose appeared, hands cradling elbows, forearms bolting her chest. Everyone was chattering except Rose. Her face was sensitive and twisted slowly to the rhythm of their words. They shuffled down the street toward Chinatown.

It was chilly outside, and we wore sweaters, my sister and me. The city seemed more in focus than during the heat of the day, each building a sharp black shape against the sky.

Rose decided to go to Utah with a family friend, stay for a while, and figure things out. Lucy informed me that Rose would come by for her things on Friday, and she didn't want me to be there. She had given Woody away to a friend.

I wrote a one-page letter, apologizing, explaining, and telling her how much I love her. My heart was a fist.

I put the letter on her bed before I left that morning. I looked around her room, vintage wallpaper now covered with artwork and posters, and felt a slow, hard ache travel from my stomach right up to my throat. I broke from its hold and ran downstairs. Stopping at the hall closet, I grabbed my neck brace and my mother's cane. I was going to be late to traffic court.

That last traffic ticket had come home to roost. If I could somehow convince the judge to dismiss it, I was home free. I had no plan. I was out of plans. I parked on a side street and walked quickly toward the courthouse until the last block, where I began my slow, phony hobble.

This judge didn't buy my story, and I was ordered to pay the fine. I gathered my props and slow-walked out of the courtroom to the cashier's window. I paid the three hundred and eighty-five dollars and walked purposefully out of the building, ripping off the neck brace as I went. It was over.

My mood had darkened by the time I pulled into the driveway a half hour later. Rose was gone. It was real now. In the afternoon, the sun moves to the back of our house, leaving the front in a deep, quiet shade. I sat down in the dreary light of the living room.

Looking down at my brown hands and forearms, I began examining the scars. Because my skin is dark, scars appear like little pale hieroglyphics. There were so many of them. That sharp little line was when I'd caught my arm on the metal mesh they use for stucco, on a job in Las Vegas. Oh, there were the two prong marks from the time I'd put the big fork right through my hand while trying to separate a frozen chicken. I'd looked away for a second and bam, got my own hand. Here's where the dog bit me when I was twelve. There were hundreds of tiny scars everywhere. A chip here, a scratch there, little crescent marks all in a row. I couldn't even identify each mishap, each assault on the surface of my body. There were too many, and it didn't matter anyway. Nothing could be done about them now.

Rose's room was a mess. It appeared that she'd rifled through all her things and hastily grabbed what she wanted. On her bed was my letter. It had been opened but left behind.

It was January, and I was sleepwalking through the winter in the grip of my misery over Rose. I hadn't heard a word from her. The days lined up, one behind the other, until it seemed she'd left long ago.

I started seeing a therapist because I was barely functioning. A gentle, smart woman about ten years my senior, she suggested I come twice a week. I liked sitting in her mid-century-style office; the sleek furniture and ethnic tapestries reminded me of my mother's house.

I poured out my story until I was drained, a brittle vessel staring across the room for help. Together, we began to sort the wreckage.

That night I had book club. I made myself go. I had to get out of my own head. Leigh was there. She had been through a grueling course of chemotherapy but was feeling better. She steadfastly maintained that she was going to kick this thing. She had so much dignity. I, on the other hand, ended up getting drunk and wallowing all over the dinner table.

The next day I called Leigh. "How bad was I?"

"Pretty bad," she said.

"I'm pathetic. I don't know why I can't snap out of this. I mean, Jesus, I got through it, and now all I can do is whine. You're still in the middle of it, and *I'm* the one making a scene."

"Listen, Mimi, you are allowed to feel dreadful. You have so much to contend with. But I have to tell you that I don't think you're doing yourself any good by indulging in self-pity. You can cry to me anytime you want, but this behavior is not helping you."

Leigh. She arrived in my life to teach me a lesson and then fly away.

My therapy took a turn. We were putting things back together now. It was a surprisingly practical process, like folding clean towels and placing them in drawers.

A few weeks later, I felt measurably better.

"Mom, Nick's here," Lucy called from downstairs.

I walked down, and he was standing in the living room with his back to me, looking into the corner. Something about his body posture was odd.

"What are you looking at, Nickboy?"

"This painting of Dad," he said. "Where is that?"

"It's Monet's garden, in Giverny. I took a picture when we were there, and then I painted it as a surprise for his birthday, remember?"

"Oh, right," he said. Then he turned around, and I could see that his eyes were filled with tears.

"Nick," I said tentatively. "Your eyes look watery. What is it?"

He shook his head in that barely perceptible way that meant there was no point in going any further. It knocked one of the tears out of his eye and down his cheek. I gave him his meds, cigarettes, and a ten-dollar bill.

"See you later, Ma."

What *was* that? What the fuck was that? Was he crying? Is that good or bad? Did I imagine it? What the hell? Looking at a picture of his father?

I knew nothing. I understood nothing.

That night I went into my studio for the first time since my operations. A row of Post-its with new painting ideas stretched across the shelf above my desk. A couple of canvases, abandoned before my first surgery, leaned against the wall. My easel stood empty, imposing . . . beckoning.

"Okay, motherfucker," I said out loud.

Paint is everywhere; every horizontal surface and even the vertical edges of my easel have all been used as a palette. I perch on my metal stool and use the area next to my haunch to mix alizarin crimson with cobalt.

The canvas I placed in front of me already had some patterns sketched out with a big brush. I try to make out what they are. It looked like people rolling on the ground. Was I seeing things that aren't there?

Not seeing things that are there?

I flick the lid off from a small jar of boiled linseed oil, dump it onto my table, and mix, mix, mix. Vandyke brown smears into Venetian red, and then there it is: the color of my son's eyes.

I'm not painting eyes, but I cover the canvas with an ocean of brown . . . rough, moving, untamed. I think of Nick asking me about Monet and then about his dad, and that tear on his face.

"What? What?" I ask his shadow. *I can't do this, Nick. Stop.*

The canvas before me starts to take form. There are mountains; there is rain; wind is blowing. Trees bend from the force of a hurricane. The sky is black.

I remember Nick leaning in toward his first love, Emily, when they were fifteen. They sat on the curb in Larchmont Village one day after school, as I drove by on my way home from the market.

My heart beating, beating, beating.

I remembered how to paint.

"**You are out** of your mind," Craig said.

"I'm doing this," I insisted.

"It's dangerous, especially in your condition."

"Bullshit. It's only dangerous if I crash and die, and that has nothing to do with my *condition*. And in case you haven't noticed, I'm back to normal. I could take *you* down, man."

"Oh my God."

"I *could*."

Craig and I had gone camping for a few days. While exploring the area, we passed a place that offered skydiving. My whole life I'd wanted to go skydiving. Craig is terrified of heights. Earlier, at our campsite, I'd seen people parachuting off the top of a towering mountain.

"I'm not going with you, Miriam," Craig warned. "If you're going to do this, you're doing it without my blessing."

"Righteo!"

When it was time to go, he said, "I'm sorry, Mimi. I can't bear it. I'll have a heart attack. I can't go."

"I know. It's fine," I said, and I headed out.

Each person was paired with an instructor and jumped in tandem. They had these contraptions where the student basically sat on the lap of the professional, so nothing could go wrong.

"Hi, I'm Cody. I'm going to be your partner," said my strapping, twenty-something teacher from Montana. I looked into his dreamy eyes as he told me the drill.

"Okay, Mimi, before we do this, let me ask you a question. Some people are thrill seekers and like to do more wild stuff, and others enjoy a placid, peaceful descent, enjoying the view. Which do you want?"

"Let's go for thrills!"

We ran steadily across the incline until Cody yelled "Now!" and we lifted our legs. It wasn't until we reached the edge that I realized how high we were. The most astounding world imaginable lay beneath us, like a painting. I was flying.

"All right," Cody yelled, "here we go!" With that we started to swoop and turn like daredevils. I was screaming. He was laughing out loud. It went on and on until finally we did a complete loop-the-loop. We began to sweep gently toward earth, the wind whispering fine new ideas in my ear. He guided us seamlessly down to a soft landing.

"I haven't done some of those moves in a long time," he said. "That was really fun. You're a trooper."

Of course I started crying and hugged him.

As I stood with my feet pressing into the earth, I marveled at the resilience of our human bodies. Cut them open, and they heal. Batter them until they turn black and blue, it always fades to that weird yellowish color and then returns to normal. Shave a head and watch the hair return. We're tough. We have two kidneys but can live with one. Take 25 percent of a person's liver for a transplant, and it grows back to full size. If this amazing body can do *that*, well, I sure as hell can heal my soul.

"I did it. I can't believe I did it!" I told Craig when I returned to our campsite.

"I know! I think I saw you," he replied.

"What do you mean? Did you follow me?"

"I climbed the hill with my binoculars," he said. "I had to make sure you didn't crash into a mountain."

"And how exactly would you have prevented *that* from the campground with your binoculars?"

"Funny." He shook his head. "How was it?"

"Craig, I was flying. I was actually flying. It was the best thing I have ever done. We did loop-the-loops!" I clapped my hands like a circus monkey.

California is a region of the earth that spans every imaginable type of terrain. Each place we visited conferred a tiny patch of healing: the skies, the grasses, the streams, the ocean. I was resuscitated by nature.

16

LONGING AND AIR

I came back from camping feeling optimistic. With no explanation at all, Rose began emailing us. She'd share experiences, send pictures, comment on what we were doing. No references to the past, though, only forward momentum.

My therapist told me I was "out of crisis," an interesting decree. I had to decide if I wanted to continue, go deeper into my childhood. We could have gone on forever, I suppose, but there were things I didn't want to look at. My perch was precarious enough, and I had no desire to spend my old age in a forensic audit of my youth. The last time I saw her we embraced, and I thanked her for rescuing me from despair.

Nick was still in his comfortable routine; there had been no bad episodes for a while. I was relieved, but every time we entered a peaceful phase I felt compelled to try something new. This schizophrenia was a train that I didn't want to stop. I didn't want it careening off a cliff somewhere, but if it pulled to a halt, that would mean it was the end of hope. I began applying to research studies.

A repeating nightmare I have is of the endless waiting rooms. Sickness is the great equalizer. I would see well-dressed, articulate parents. There were also people who looked like they lived on the street. Every type was represented—suits, uniforms, work boots, sweats. We all sat and waited. We all had the same complaint: nothing ever worked. We'd fill out all the papers, over and over. Then we would smile because we knew getting annoyed only made things worse. The person on the other side of the desk held our fates.

Filling out the applications was a particularly painful thing for me. It was an official reminder of what was wrong with Nick.

- *Does the patient have a job?* NO
- *Does the patient have children?* NO
- *Does the patient drive?* NO
- *Does the patient take medications for his condition?* YES
- *Does the patient smoke?* YES
- *Does the patient consume alcohol?* YES
- *If so, how much?* WHO KNOWS?
- *Can the patient prepare his own food?* YES
- *Did I ever imagine, in my wildest dreams, that I'd need to clarify whether my adult son could make a sandwich?* NO

I remember the dashing younger Nick, carefully cleaning the old car his granddad had given to him. He'd put on a vintage bowling shirt with *Steve* embroidered over the pocket and head out to bulldog chicks. I could see his thick sweep of hair, brushed back and shining. The girls eyed him. The guys looked up to him.

Let us stay there. That time.

The same year he got the car, we went to a Christmas party at Laura's house. He arrived separately, with his crew. I'd decided to get dressed up for a change. I was wearing a sleeveless gray satin dress that was cut on the bias, so it swirled as I walked.

"Mom! You look really beautiful," he stated. "I mean it. You look beautiful."

That's the boy I want. Each time I had to fill out a questionnaire it reminded me, unmercifully, that *that* Nick was gone. He was never going to get married. He was never going to be a father. I hated Questionnaire Nick.

- *Does he have friends?*   NO
- *Does he have a future?*   NO

As suddenly as she had appeared, Rose went off the radar again. No emails. I enlisted a network of her friends to keep track of her. I had my brother make a fake Facebook profile for me. Methodically, I began friending her friends so I might get a glimpse of her page or a mention of her somewhere. I sat at night, scouring through other people's photo sections, searching for that Modigliani face of hers.

"Lucy, come here," I called. "It's important!"

"What, Ma?" She flopped on the daybed.

"No, come here, look!"

"What is it?" She slowly got up.

"Look, look here at this picture. In the background, is that Rose?"

"Oh my God, Mom, you have to stop . . ."

"No, look closely. I think it's her."

"It's a shadow," Lucy replied with disdain.

I couldn't argue with that.

Running into Nick's friends was always hard. They were all getting older now, out of college and into adult life. In the early years, his close friends had tried to maintain contact, but it was difficult. Now he was in another world altogether. The chasm between them had become a bridge too far. They were becoming doctors and lawyers, getting married; Nick spent the majority of his waking hours watching TV.

"I just saw a cool show, Mom. Did you know that when you get struck by lightning your shoes fly off?"

It was so hard not to compare, measure where he should have

been. I'd lay his tattered outline over their big, full lives and mourn.

I fashioned a strategy to deal with the absence of Rose. She had screamed at me, in one of the last fights we had, that she felt invisible. I thought, *What if I just start emailing the memories I have of her?* Proof that she had been seen, loved? I wrote down the story of when she toddled down the middle of Norton Avenue in her diaper, like Swee'Pea in the Popeye cartoons, so oblivious to danger that it never touched her. I felt slightly better as I pressed *Send*.

I'd found a support group for young people with mental illness. It was all the way in Culver City, but it sounded good. I went to tell Nick. He stood, leaning against his building, smoking, looking rather cool.

"Hey, Bub, how are you doing?" I asked.

"Sure," he replied.

"Sure? *Sure* is how you're doing?" I just couldn't help myself.

Nothing.

"Never mind. Listen, I found a good group meeting for you to go to. It's tomorrow night. I'll drive you."

"I don't know. Let's think about it for a while."

I offered to buy him dinner afterward, and he agreed to go. The group met at 5:30 p.m., so we were smack in the middle of rush hour. It took forty-five minutes to get there. I had to let him control the radio in the car so he'd stay calm. This meant a playlist of weird stuff from Ranchero to New Age to an electronic assault that didn't even sound like music. As we pulled up, I put on a big smile and said, "Here we are! This is going to be great."

I sat in the Starbucks down the street and composed another email to Rose. I told her the story about getting measles when I was pregnant with her. I'd caught it from the other kids and worried for the rest of the pregnancy that it had hurt her.

"So. How was the meeting?" I asked before he was even all the way into the car.

"Fine."

I asked more questions, but that was all I got. At least he'd attended and agreed to continue. When I was finally home, I went through the mail. It was all the usual stuff. From the pile, a creamy, small envelope fell out. It was an invitation to Nick's old friend Jack's wedding. It smelled like baby powder.

I remembered how, when Rose was an infant, nursing, she would reach her tiny arm out and pat me. Over and over, on the side of my back. I sent her an email telling her how wonderful that had been.

The weeks went by. I had no idea what went on in those meetings. I was trying to pull back on the micromanaging.

"So, Nick, Jack's wedding is next week. Have you thought about it? Do you want to go?" I asked after a meeting.

"I don't think so," he said. I didn't even want to go. A big event filled with the personifications of everything Nick had lost—just what I needed. But Bridget and Jack were like family. I had to rise above my shitty emotions.

That night I wrote to Rose about the way she used to dress up like a hobo when all the other girls wanted to be princesses.

Jack's wedding was on a Saturday afternoon at his house on Ridgewood Place. I felt a tug for the carefree days we'd spent there. They set up chairs on the front lawn; the porch was to serve as the stage. Bridget is a musician and had a sweet collection of her fellow artists performing. Groups of strapping young men and lovely girls milled around, waiting for the ceremony. I looked for Bridget.

I managed to congratulate her with a big, fixed smile, although a lump was developing in my throat. I talked to Jack and met his bride. As the ceremony began, I found myself backing off the lawn, standing on the sidewalk. Then I ran off, over the familiar cracked cement where tree roots had broken through, and back to my car. As I pulled away, I noticed how green the leaves were at that time of day. Otherworldly.

Sprawled on my daybed, still in my fancy dress, I was ashamed. I had wanted to be brave and happy for Jack. But I wasn't. I hated him.

I thought about my mother at the potter's wheel. The essential part of being able to throw pots is the centering of the clay. One must be able to place it exactly in the middle. There is no shortcut. I'd see her sitting there, effortlessly forming one lump of clay after another into bowls. She tried to teach me, but I never got it. I faked it. I'd jam my hand against the clay, my elbow into my rib cage, and force it. You *can* produce some pottery that way. But a keen eye knows a bowl that has been centered properly, and my mother called me on it, over and over.

"But it looks fine, Ma. What's the difference?"

"The difference is integrity."

A couple of times I got it. That simple, perfect place that is center. It was different from anything else. It felt like flying. Carefully, precisely, you pull the piece into shape. The slightest unintended movement could send it a million miles back to wrong. It's not like painting, where you can splash pigment over mistakes; throwing pots is an endeavor of absolutes.

The last conversation I'd had with my mother was a stupid fight over the phone. I didn't call her for two days. I even drove right by her apartment the second day but didn't stop. Later, I realized she must have been lying on the floor that day, unable to move because of the stroke.

She never regained consciousness.

The secret is that she *did*. I swear to God, alone with me in the emergency room, she spoke. Everyone else was outside. I leaned over and asked her, "Ma, can you hear me?" She exhaled slowly. "Yessss." Now I wonder if I imagined it. I can still hear that "Yessss" late at night when I am alone. I wrote to Rose and told her this.

I put on my worst sweatpants and raggedy T-shirt. I needed a friend, and fast.

"Brooke, get me out of here. I'm circling the drain." I held the phone like it was hot.

"What's going on?" she asked.

"Oh, it was Jack's wedding today, and I was a big fat infant and left, and now I hate myself and can't stop thinking about my mother and what a fake I am."

"That's not good. I'm about to take the dogs out. Why don't you come to the canyon with me?"

"Not a damn hike! I hate hikes."

"It would be good for you, Mimi. Come on, I'll pick you up."

"I was thinking more like a whole lot of food and binge-watching Netflix."

It was delightful in the park. We got to the top just as the sun went down.

"You're right, I feel better," I said, once I got control of my breath.

"It's nice, right?"

"I can't believe you do this every day. You're insane."

"You should bring Buster and do it with me."

"What would I do without my Brookie?" I asked, and hugged her.

I went home and wrote to Rose about the sky. I reminisced about the time I had to stuff gauze in her leg. I promised her I would always love her. As always, I felt a slight shiver of static as I pressed *Send*.

The next Thursday I drove Nick to his meeting. "So how are the meetings going, Nick?" I asked.

"They're nice."

The traffic was particularly bad that evening. As we sat in grid-lock, he turned to me and said, "Do you know what a green room is?"

"What do you mean?"

"You know, late night."

"Oh," I said, suddenly getting it, "you mean where they wait to go on the talk shows?"

"Yeah."

"Yeah, I know what that is. What about them?"

"Nothing. I was just thinking about them." He turned away to the window as the light changed from red to green.

I dropped him off and headed up to Starbucks. The place was jammed, nowhere to sit. *Screw it*, I thought, *I'm going to Johnnie's Pastrami and having me a meal*. The way to Johnnie's was back down Sepulveda, right past the mental health center. I'd have time. As I passed, I saw Nick, sitting on some steps down from the building, smoking. I pulled a fast U-turn and jumped out of the car.

"Nick! What are you doing out here?"

"Um, having a cigarette," he said.

"But the meeting just started. Why would they break already?"

He just stared blankly at me. Things were starting to come together in my head. I brushed past him and walked into the building to find out. They told me Nick left the first meeting midway and never attended again. I had been driving through awful traffic every Thursday, wasting time, buying him dinner, for weeks, for nothing.

Enraged, I stormed out of the office. "Get in the car."

He lumbered over and got in the passenger seat. I took off like a race car driver.

"What the fucking hell, Nick? Really? You haven't been going to the meetings all this time?"

"No," he said simply.

"No? No, what? No, I haven't been going to the meetings? No, I have?"

"Mom, don't overreact."

"Nick, I want the truth."

Crickets.

"I know you have not gone to a single meeting since the first night. I just talked to the lady in charge."

He just sat there. Once or twice he'd shake his head slightly, but he didn't say a word. I threatened him with all kinds of punishments and reductions in his rations, but the truth was, there wasn't any way to give him a consequence. I was the payee for his SSDI money, and it just covered his rent. We gave him ten dollars and a pack of cigarettes a day. That had been the original deal when he agreed to take his meds years before. If I threatened to take that away, he'd always point it out.

He had a bed, a table, a chair, and a television with basic cable. A couple of times a year we'd get him a few pairs of the same corduroy pants and the black T-shirts he wore every day. He was unpunishable.

I pulled up in front of his building and said softly, "Just get out."

He quietly stood, closed the door, and walked toward his place.

That night I wrote to Rose and apologized for not seeing her, for becoming a ghost, for not being the mother the other kids had had. I told her that I understood why she was angry.

An envelope arrived containing a tax return check for Rose. From my sleuthing, I knew she'd reached the East Coast and was out of money. I'd gotten a report from one of my operatives that she was sleeping in Central Park with friends. I hadn't heard her voice in more than three months. This was my chance! I texted immediately.

"I have some money of yours that you might want."

Five minutes later: "What are you talking about?"

"If you're interested, call me on the phone." I realized this might be my one chance.

I was at the paint store, praying for the phone to ring. She wasn't taking the bait. Damn. Finally, it rang.

"Hello?" I said, trying to sound normal.

"Hi. It's me." Her voice. Her voice!

"Hi, Rose. What's up?"

"Well, you said you have some money of mine. What's that about?"

"Oh, I guess it's a tax refund. I thought you might want it." It took all I had to stay even.

"Yeah, actually, that would be great," she said.

"So, what do you want me to do?"

We discussed the logistics, figured it out, and I said, tentatively,

"How are you doing?"

"Great. My friends are assholes, and I'm all alone now." *Tell me where you are! I'll be on the next plane! I'll rock you in my arms.*

"That sucks. Anything I can do?" Cool as a cucumber.

"No, not really. But thanks for sending me the money. That will help."

"Okay, Rose. It's good to hear your voice. Keep in touch."

"Thanks, Mom." Click.

I stood in that dreary strip mall, filled with joy and grief all tangled up into one ghastly emotion. I smelled exhaust and, for some reason, frying chicken.

Leigh was undergoing another round of chemo. Her cancer was doggedly hanging on—the son of a bitch wouldn't let go. All us gals set up a support system for her, took her to doctors' appointments, visited regularly. We bathed her; we changed her sheets. She held court from the massive bed in her living room. We brought her the most nutritious food and then ate it ourselves because she had no appetite. We sprawled like figures in the Manet picnic, all over her bed, and mused about the past. She was going down, but nobody said a word.

The summer was crushing in Los Angeles; the nights held the heat, making it impossible to sleep. I decided to escape to Washington for a while. We had put in a garden, and the flowers would be coming in about now. Craig worked on the house, and I painted and did thousand-piece jigsaw puzzles. It was kind of horrible, nowhere to look but at the truth and at the trees. I might as well have stayed in therapy.

One day in mid-August, the constant harbinger of happiness and woe rang.

"Ma, it's Lucy. Guess what?"

Does my blood run cold or do I jump for joy?

"Rose called! They're on their way to LA!"

They. "Who is they?" I asked.

"She's with Shannon and her boyfriend, and I think Rose's boyfriend too."

Rose has a boyfriend?

"She can come home now, right? I mean, I know Dad threw her out, but she can come home now?"

I was scared and thrilled at the same time. "When will they be there?"

"Tomorrow!"

"Let me talk to Dad, and I'll call you back."

I squatted next to Craig on the porch, one elbow on the arm of his chair. "What should we do?" I asked as a light rain fell.

"What do you mean?"

"Well, you threw her out. The ball is kind of in your court."

"Mimi, she's our daughter. I know what I did, but it was at a time of incredible stress. It's her home. Of course she is welcome there." He straightened up in the chair and turned to face me.

I jumped up, ran in, and called Lucy. "Of course she can come home!" There was no direct communication between Rose and me.

"I guess we should go down there," Craig said, walking in and taking off his jacket. Blades of grass floated to the floor.

"Listen. I need to ask you for something," I said tentatively. "I want to go down first. Alone. It's been months since I've seen her, spoken to her, and I want a week alone to reconnect. Can you give me that?"

"What, I'm not welcome in my own home?" *Here we go.*

"No. It is not that. I've been in a state of complete anguish for all these months. I want my time. I need to reconnect with her by myself. Please give this to me." I stood in front of him, my bare feet wet.

He agreed to wait.

I walked up the variegated stone steps we'd put in the year we bought the house. I had a small overnight bag and a whole lot of apprehension. I was about to see the child I'd ached for, agonized over, for months. She was in her room with the flowered wallpaper. As my key turned in the door, I recalled other days, days when a throng of little children would come running at that sound, shouting, "Mom's home! Mom's home!"

Today, silence.

Rose's door was the first on the left. It was closed. I knocked.

"Rose," I said softly.

"Yeah. Come in."

Opening the door, I saw a room scattered with clothing, musical instruments, something that looked like a goat hide, and a tattooed boy sprawled on the bed. Rose stood nearby. I couldn't contain myself; I went directly to her, wrapped my arms around her, and for the first time in months, I felt peace.

Over the week, Rose and I tentatively, cautiously, moved toward each other. I asked nothing of her.

Mother love—it rushes through our veins, escapes sometimes in the form of salt water at the intersection of eyelids and the edge underneath, but it will never leave us. There is no real exit. It doesn't wane, mother love. It lives in the body, the corporeal residence of grief, loss, and joy. All this commotion might reside in my heart. Or in a fingernail, or my lower back. Who knows? But this I know for sure: I hold it in my body. The same body that grew them.

Over and over, we send that love out there like a folded paper boat, which will, incongruously, float merrily along for a while. Water, which devours paper, plays along. But eventually it nibbles at the bottom edge of the construct, reminding us of the truth of the physical world. Tomorrow, when you walk by the pond, a puff of mush will lie, unseen, at the bottom.

But even that doesn't change a thing.

Mother love.

After a week, Craig returned. He and Rose had a warm reunion, no problems there.

That evening, after dinner, Craig and I sat on the back porch talking.

"So, how is Nick?" Craig asked.

"Still crazy."

"Why didn't he come up tonight?"

"He seemed really out of it this morning when I went down there. I called all afternoon, but no answer. Just one of those days."

"Lucy told me he hangs out at Safeway all night. He made friends with a guy there who gives him the leftover samples," Craig said.

We sat listening to the thump of Buster's tail.

"Miriam," Craig said quietly.

"Yeah?"

"A father's love is different from a mother's love."

"What?" We were both looking at the liquidambar tree.

"I know you think I've abandoned Nick, but you know what it is, don't you?"

Now I looked at him.

"I've always felt a little different . . . growing up, being an artist. I mean, now everyone is an artist, but it wasn't that way when we were growing up. I was the weird kid, Miriam. There isn't anything I can do to make Nick not schizophrenic."

"Craig, what are you saying? I'm not following."

"The reason I can't look at Nick is that I feel like I am just a hair's breadth away from being just like him."

I looked at my hands, always with splotches of paint on them, big and bony. Craig just continued to stare at the tree. We sat there, together, until it got dark and a dim flicker of stars dotted the night.

The next day, Rose's boyfriend boarded a bus to Maine to visit his parents. Their plan was to meet back in New Orleans.

Leigh was disappearing in front of our eyes. We planned one last get-together at the beach house. Though nobody came right out and said it, we knew it was our swan song.

It was a time. We took walks, played games, smoked pot, begged Leigh to share her pain meds with us. It was winter, but it was California and we were at the beach, so Carolyn and I braved the cold water. The others said we were reckless. We were pleased to be reckless. We were pleased to be alive. There is a photograph of us all that looks like it was taken by Annie Leibovitz—not because it looks professional, but because it shows the truth of all the love and fear in the universe.

Back in LA, I took Nick to his local El Pollo Loco for lunch. We waited in a long line. I stood by as he gave his detailed order. He quietly went over to the salsa bar to serve up more tiny plastic bowls than he could eat in a year.

"You are his mother?" the woman behind the counter asked me.

"Yes, I am," I said, imagining some nuisance created by his frequent visits.

Her eyes got soft, and she put her hand over mine on the Formica. "I am so glad to know he has a mother. He is a good boy. He has manners."

I couldn't speak. I looked at her with my own misty eyes and nodded slowly.

Before we left, I went back to the counter. "Does he come here a lot?"

"Oh, yes, a few times a week. Don't you worry. We all watch over him."

I left the restaurant, held together only by longing and air.

17

MOON COMING

Lucy was restless. Living at home after college had not been the plan.

"Mom, I want to lose some weight. What do I do?" she asked me one day.

"Why? You look great."

"Well, I've gained about ten pounds since college, and I want to take it off. It's not a big deal. I just want to," she said sensibly.

I told her the best way, in my opinion, was to just lower her consumption of food and add more exercise. It was a simple, no-fail formula.

Nick was more engaged than he'd been in a while and came up to the house almost every night for dinner. The last time I'd cleaned his apartment, I had to throw away all the art supplies I'd bought him. They were on the kitchen counter in a half inch of water, melting into a useless pile of colorful sludge.

A drawing pad was on the table, saved from a soggy demise. It had been sitting there for months, untouched. It was open to the last entry, a series of scribbles. There were some pictures but mostly a lot of lists and fractured thoughts, written out in cursive. I went to the first page.

> art class
>
> show
>
> catering
>
> computer
>
> bike
>
> car

That, I understood completely. These were things he was going to do to get his life back on track. He must have written it quite a while ago.

> Well, I hope to see improvement. I run to God. Run to
> mannered obstinance, aware not to depend on my speculations
> and dreams. I breathe and enjoy what's given. Simplicity,
> happiness, and laughter at facade, parts played, roles, and
> reverse psychology.

I wanted to stop reading. I didn't want to be privy to this, but I felt it was incumbent on me to visit his world, at least try to understand. I couldn't afford to overlook anything, because the answer might be anywhere.

> if there would ever be a way to die
> it might be a two bird stone slippery dagger, dribble drabble shaky
> white t-shirt
> absorbent blanketing
> guishing
> That was yesteryear
> I'm a timber wolf.

It was getting harder to stick with it.

> When all the phones are off the hook
> all the bubble wrap's been
> popped
> There's nothing left to do but
> Beat the pillows with celery sticks

My stomach was physically cramping. I didn't know the person who had written those words. I took the pad home with me.

"Mom, I've been doing what you said for three weeks now, and I haven't lost a pound," Lucy complained one night.

"Really? Are you sure you have been strict?" I asked.

"Yeah. I don't get it."

"Well, if that's the case, you should make an appointment with your doctor just to make sure everything's good. I mean, I'm sure it's nothing, but if you've been following the diet, you should have lost some weight by now."

I often wondered what had become of Nick's paintings. I assumed he'd taken them up to Washington and abandoned them there. I dreamed of them occasionally, scattered like quilts along the West Coast with his other missing belongings. The thought of that was excruciatingly painful for me. It was in his art that I could still locate him. As his disease progressed, his art making wandered. His old work held the boy I knew—clear, articulate brushstrokes painted with the certainty of a venerable artist.

And then, cleaning out our storage sheds one day, I found them. Like a frantic archaeologist urgently unhoarding a major dig, I pulled painting after painting out into the driveway. I lined all the canvases up along the side of the house. I couldn't believe they had been there all along. I was sweating, even though it was cool out. My heart seemed to move slightly higher in my chest, beating against my sternum.

Bright palette, strong strokes of movement, unsettling combustion of realistic and abstract. All in one place, his work created a wallop of beauty that brought me to my knees. Large canvases of dense, brilliant Kandinsky-like abstraction. Smaller, ironic, intellectual studies of color and shape. Strange, disconcerting female bodies . . . sexual and evocative. Pristine figurative portraits, perfectly rendered. It was the body of work of a lifetime painted in a few short years of adolescence. How could this be? How could this have happened, that the boy who painted like a master was just gone? I walked up and down the driveway, talking out loud.

"Look at these! Look at these paintings! How in this derelict world is it possible that he is gone?"

Lowering down onto the cold driveway, I rolled to my side, weeping. I could feel the aggregate pressing into my cheek, the stones, their edges. And I floated back to a memory of my childhood, when I fell on the ragged rock path in our yard the day before first grade. I had to walk into the class with a scabby, scary-looking lacerated mouth and face. I was a freak, an outlier, before I even knew that word.

Lying on the gray cement, it felt like there was nowhere in the world for me and my son.

I was so happy, grateful that I'd found the paintings. I went inside with the intention of doing something about it. But what? Hours passed, and eventually I went back out and put all the paintings carefully back into the shed.

I felt like I had found him. Nick lived safely in those paintings.

A few days later, I was at a party in the neighborhood. We'd all known each other for so long, watched our children grow, seen the facades we created crumble into truth. With the correct combination of alcohol and abandon, things could get very real. I was talking to my friend Melanie. I told her about the paintings.

"Mimi, you should have a show. People should see his work."

"Oh, I don't know. Where would I do it? How would I do it?"

"Let's do it at Busby's!" Busby's was the restaurant she and her husband owned.

"Oh, I couldn't ask you to do that."

"You're not asking me—I'm suggesting it," she said. "Let me talk to Paul. I think this could be great."

"Melanie, if you mean it, I'm going to take you up on this, so are you sure you mean it?" I was already starting to have grandiose ideas.

"I am completely serious."

We began the grand scheme of Nick's entry into the art world, the public eye. We'd stage a huge opening, get a lot of press relating mental illness and the potential for hope. It would be wonderful for Nick and would create buzz for the restaurant as well. Nick would start painting again!

I presented the idea to Nick.

"Okay," he said. "I'll do it."

Melanie and I met a few times. A date was set. We planned our strategy to get press coverage. Nick would be recognized as the prodigy he was. It could lead to monetary and critical success, and that would be a path to a cure. Someone would step forward with a groundbreaking treatment. Certainly, the resurrection of such a talent would inspire the finest minds of science. The tableau began to take shape in my mind.

A couple of weeks later, Nick and I sat at Sizzler, his favorite place. The fantastic thing about that restaurant was the impossible array of incongruous foods.

"So, Bub, we're on track for this show of yours. Are you stoked?"

"Sure."

"It's going to be great. You could make some real money selling your work."

"You mean the paintings would be for sale?"

"Of course. It's an art show."

"You mean other people would have my paintings in their houses?" he asked.

Oh, no.

"Yeah, that's how it works. It'll be great." My throat constricted, and this came out like a squeak.

Nick did the slow head shake. "I don't know if I want my paintings in people's houses."

"What do you mean?"

"Well, I'm not sure about this. I don't think I want the paintings to be out of the shed."

As so often in the past, I paused in a desperate attempt to make him see how this would benefit him. Didn't we all long for him and his work to be enjoyed and appreciated? What, I ransacked my mind, could I say to secure this for him, from him? "Nick, I have put a lot of time into this. So has Melanie. I cannot let these people put time and energy into this if you are going to back out." I wanted to sweep the salad bar across the restaurant with my left arm and toss the table through the window with my right.

"I don't want to do this, Mom," he said resolutely. "Tell them forget it."

I placed my fork softly next to the crazy assortment of food on my plate. I took a deep breath. What had I been thinking? That some fancy *art show* had the power to mitigate the grim, sabotaging reality of the schizophrenia? I picked up my fork and divided my attention between the carnitas and seafood macaroni salad. Nick sat contentedly across from me, oblivious to the carnage in my soul.

We drove home without a word. I left him at his building and began driving up to our house. Before I had traveled two blocks, he called me.

"Ma. You forgot to give me my cigarettes."

"Okay. Wait outside," I replied in a monotone. God dammit. Just when I think I'm out, I'm called back. And it's my own fault. I forgot to give him the cigarettes, so I had to turn the corner, drive back down to Ninth Street, and face my insane son one more time.

I pulled up to his front door and opened my window. I handed him a pack of cigarettes.

"See ya later, Ma," he said sweetly.

"Yeah. Bye, Nickboy."

That night I was alone in the house. I retired to my studio and opened a bottle of wine. I watched television. I painted. I implored the heavens to cut this shit out. I googled Nicholas O'Rourke on my computer. He didn't exist in the cyber world. His birth certificate was in the safety deposit box at the bank; that was proof on paper. I spent the rest of the night looking at other Nicholas O'Rourkes on the internet and seeing what their lives were like. I awoke on the daybed in the morning, still in my clothes.

Melanie was very gracious, which made it worse. I had my own exhibition coming up at Leigh's gallery, so I decided to concentrate on that for a while. I had been looking forward to it for so long. I permitted myself this anticipation and immersed myself in this, my own art—not a commissioned mural or something for someone else. This was mine.

Nick's paintings rested for years in the storage shed until, in an act of solitary restitution, I hung them all in the stairway to my studio. Salon style, from the floor to the ceiling.

Lucy had gone to get a physical, and the doctor said she seemed fine. All her blood work had come back normal. She was just going to have to try a little harder on the diet thing. The doctor had found a little lump in her throat and ordered a sonogram. She told her that it might be a small cyst. We got Lucy one of those small trampolines she could keep in her room, thinking that ought to get her metabolism up.

Leigh died. I was able to have my bedside farewell with her, tell her how much she meant to me, thank her for being such a fine friend.

The irony of Leigh's death in relation to my life tapped away at my consciousness. She'd had the brain tumor at a time when I didn't know her well. Then I got the same thing, and she waltzed onto center stage in my life.

Then she got cancer. Soon, I was the healthy friend trying to soften her descent. I'd never stayed by someone through the process of dying. When my father died, I was young and pretended it wasn't happening. My mother's stroke and death haunted me. My weird sense of duty about Leigh had puzzled me at the time. Once she died, it dawned on me: I'd been a coward with both of my parents. I had needed to do this because I loved Leigh, but also because it was my opportunity to stand in the fire. I showed myself that I could do it. She'd suffered terribly, with dignity and strength. Now she was dead, and I was alive. I vowed to myself that I would live more graciously. I moved more deeply into my yoga practice. I tried to be nicer to people.

"Mom, the doctor said that I have a growth on my thyroid. She says that they're really common, and she's sure it's nothing, but they want to do a biopsy," Lucy announced.

"Are you sure?" My hand gripped the steering wheel like I was hanging from it.

"Yeah, it's really no big deal. She says they just want to make sure. I'm going in on Thursday."

"Well, I'm taking you."

"No, Mom. It's nothing. It only takes about five minutes." She was firm.

My knuckles were a pale unhealthy color, cerulean blue cut with titanium white.

When Lucy was four, she developed a routine we all found fascinating. For some unknown reason, every day at dusk, she'd run around the whole house frantically closing all the curtains and blinds. She didn't seem scared or particularly upset. She just scurried around shouting, "Moon coming! Moon coming!" Craig and I watched with bemusement. She was such a little bundle of delight.

Sitting at the desk in my office, I admired the view. It must have originally been a sleeping porch—windows lined two walls. I'd measured them for curtains, and all eight windows varied in size. No two were the same; one was almost two inches bigger than the others. I could see the row of homes behind us. The sky was washed in deep colors, and my tall liquidambar tree stood in all its October glory, cascading falls of ochre, umber, and chromium green. Rose was in her room working on music when I heard the front door open.

"Luce, is that you?" I called.

I heard her walking quickly up the stairs and turned to see her march into the room holding her phone to her ear, a stricken look on her face.

"I . . . can't." She held the phone out to me.

"Hello? This is Lucy's mother. Who is this, please?"

"Oh, hello. This is Dr. Ajamian at Kaiser. I was just giving Lucy the results of her biopsy. I will need her permission to speak with you. Can you please put her back on the line?"

The ligature of terror took hold of me as I handed the phone back to Lucy. "I have cancer," she said, her green eyes welling up like they used to when she was little. She managed to give the doctor permission before dissolving onto the daybed.

Rose walked into the room just as Lucy said "cancer." She stood there, motionless.

By now I could shift into crisis mode in the blink of an eye. I had a ten-minute conversation with Dr. Ajamian, asked all the appropriate questions, and jotted down her answers. An appointment was set for the following day.

Sitting next to Lucy, I held her in my arms. She'd stopped crying, but the expression on her face was a terrible combination of disbelief and fright—like a strange rag doll.

"It's going to be okay, Lulu," I said with certainty. "Let me tell you what the doctor said."

She rocked back and forth, arms crossed, moaning.

"Thyroid cancer is one of the most treatable cancers there is. They've found just a small tumor, and it doesn't seem to have spread at all. You are going to be fine. Fine. They will remove it, and your life will be fine." I really had to shut up before I said "fine" one more time.

"What do we do?" she asked quietly.

"We will go see Dr. Ajamian tomorrow and decide on a course of action. This is not even life-threatening, babydoll. We're going to get you through this. Right, Rose?"

Rose was still standing, oddly reminiscent of a statue of St. Francis of Assisi I'd seen once, staring at us. Her palms were at her sides, opening forward. At the sound of her name, she reanimated and came to sit.

"Sure. Mom's right. The doctor said."

"Okay, then I am going to believe you." She took a deep breath. "But, Mom, I don't want you telling everyone about this like you always do with everything."

"Lucy, this isn't something to be embarrassed about. You are going to need your friends' support."

"It's not that. I just don't want to be *Cancer Girl*. I don't want everyone in Larchmont looking at me with pity. I'll decide who I tell."

I stopped in my tracks, benumbed by the question of what I had taught her by my own behavior.

Rose offered to take her out and get her mind off it. Lucy and I hugged like lovers, not enough limbs to demonstrate our devotion.

I had to tell Craig. I called his cell. Straight to voice mail. I turned to the internet, filled with information sufficient to scare myself to death.

For about an hour I alternated between reading every gruesome fact about thyroid cancer and calling Craig repeatedly. Between what I was finding out and my frustration trying to reach Craig, I began to crumble.

Where was he? Why couldn't I reach him? He was always reachable. Had something unimaginable happened to him as well? Was he lying dead somewhere from another atrial infarction? Lucy had cancer. Lucy had CANCER.

I began to gulp for air—the harder I tried, the less oxygen I got. I calmed myself down enough to realize I had to call a friend. I called Brenda. No answer. I called Brooke. No answer. I called every friend I had, and not one person answered the phone. I couldn't believe it. I have a million friends. Where the hell was everybody? Still no Craig. Lucy and Rose were evidently making a night of it. The phone rang at about nine. It was Carolyn.

"Mimi, I was watching Obama's speech, and I took out my phone and saw you'd called a bunch of times. Are you okay?" Oh. Obama's speech.

The floodgates opened. After the psychotic journey I'd been on, I lost it at the sound of a concerned human voice.

"It's Lucy. It's cancer," I wailed. "This can't be happening. Not Lucy. How can this be happening?"

"Hang on. Just hang on. I'll be right there," she said.

Grabbing at the banister like person having a seizure, I went downstairs. Crying so hard I was still having trouble breathing, I stumbled out onto the front porch where I curled up and waited for Carolyn.

"What can I do? What do you need?" Carolyn called out as she ran up the walkway.

"I don't know," I cried. "I don't know what to do."

She sat with me on the steps and listened to my convoluted story. I went on and on about how it couldn't be true. *Where was Craig?* I couldn't take any more. I wasn't strong enough.

"All right," she said evenly. "Let's get you inside."

We went up to my bedroom. The warm incandescent light on my nightstand threw a halo of gold on the pillow.

"Do you want anything to drink? Eat?" she asked.

I knew exactly what I wanted.

"Put me to bed. I want to go to bed. In the bathroom, top drawer in the middle, sleeping pills. Bring me two. Then please unplug the phone and sit with me until I fall asleep. Lock the door when you leave. If the girls come home while you're here, tell them I was just super tired."

Carolyn did as I asked. The last thing I remember was her lying next to me and rubbing my back, just like a mother does with a child after a nightmare.

The next day I was back in control. The girls had come home late and knew nothing of my breakdown. I made up my mind: my daughter had cancer, and she was not going to get Broken Mom. I called Craig, who had been at a friend's house the night before with no cell reception. We didn't even bother with the *how can this be happening?* We just exchanged facts and made plans. He'd fly home the next day.

As we were leaving for Kaiser, Nick showed up. I looked at Lucy. "What do you want to do?"

"Just tell him."

"Nick, we have some bad news, but it's going to be all right. It turns out that Lucy has thyroid cancer. But she's going to have an operation and have it removed."

"So she'll be fine, then?"

"Yes, she will."

"Okay, do you have my cigarettes?"

"Go inside and tell Rose I said to give them to you. We have to go."

"Well, that was traumatic," Lucy said as we got in the car.

As I watched the soft-spoken doctor knead my daughter's throat, feeling with sensitive fingers the tissue below, I felt oddly serene. It was the almost loving way this doctor touched her.

I had spent a lot of time in hospitals over the last few years. When my mother was in the coma and we brought the children to say goodbye, a nurse had rushed in ahead of us to make her look nice. We all stared at my mother with her hair styled like a little girl's. The tender intelligence of the nurses, who wash sick bodies and dress wounds, tells them when to comfort and when to stand back.

We discussed all the options and decided that Lucy would have her whole thyroid removed. She'd have to take medication for the rest of her life, but it was the only way to eliminate any possibility of the cancer returning. We scheduled yet another surgery.

Everybody went about their business and didn't discuss Lucy's cancer. Something had shifted position in my psyche with this turn of events. I went to work, interacted with clients, even contacted several mental health facilities about new opportunities for Nick, but my insides were like a flurry of bark dust in a wood chipper. My internal organs, my brain, my heart, my memories—all shredded. Shredded and whirling like a savage tornado, pushing from the inside out with its relentless thrust.

I just watched TV all the time. I had settled on a hideous movie on Lifetime about a woman who had inadvertently killed her son. He was four years old. She took his body and buried it in the woods. Digging the grave, she told herself that she was making his bed one last time. In the scene where she finally confessed, she began to howl. Deep, guttural, primal sounds. She threw herself against the walls and at the furniture. The policeman tried to restrain her. It was impossible. A bunch of men came into the room. Two held her arms, two held her legs, one stood at her head as she tried to bash it against something. Did it take five men? Did it take ten, twenty men? How many men did it take to hold her grief and contain her pain? A hundred men at each limb, a cold steel vise at her skull—nothing would be enough to contain that woman's anguish, her bottomless grief.

I watched the movie, and I thought, *That is me, one cellophane-slim measure away from being a howling animal.*

As Craig and I drove Lucy to the hospital for her surgery, deeply roughed autumn leaves scattered, making staccato rhythms on the asphalt. She was stoic and composed. "I just want to get it over with," she said when I tried to give her an encouraging little speech.

As they prepared her for surgery, she asked, "Did you know that Nick used to knock on my door, late, after you'd gone to sleep? He'd play me the newest song he'd taught himself on his guitar. He'd sit on the hallway bench and serenade me. It was so sweet. I wish he was here now."

"I'll bring him over tonight so you can visit," Craig said.

"Mom. Dad. Nick is the person who molded me into who I am today. I wouldn't know anything about anything if it weren't for him." Her eyes shined with urgency; her jaw was tight.

"He loves you very much, Lucy." I touched her cheek.

"No. It's more than that!" Her face became heated. "He showed me the way to live. With art. With music. And he didn't do it for any other reason than to just have me know. Because he knew, and he wanted me to understand the beauty also." Her eyes, magnified by tears, were something you could just fall into.

I realized then that the keen cut of Nick's loss would be with her always, just like the tiny Basquiat's crown she had tattooed on her outer right wrist—because Nick had introduced her to his work.

We were told it would be two to three hours, and the doctor would come find us in the surgery waiting room. Rose showed up, then Sara. We watched TV and cracked a lot of inappropriate jokes. Craig dozed off at one point. For two hours and fifty minutes, I was fine. It wasn't a risky surgery. They'd take it out, and she would recover. The last ten minutes I hung on, but as soon as we reached the three-hour mark, I went berserk. The clock on the wall began to tick loudly, like in an old black-and-white noir movie. The scraping of someone moving a chair sounded deafening. Craig was leafing through a magazine, the pages flapping like the sail on a boat. Sara and Rose seemed to be hollering at each other for some reason.

"Craig!" I whispered. "It's been *over* three hours. Something is wrong. I know something is wrong!" I no longer had any capacity to trust in a good outcome.

"It's okay. They said the time was approximate. It could have taken longer to get her into the operating room."

What was wrong with everyone? They all just sat there like it wasn't obvious that Lucy had died. I crossed my arms in front of my chest and held on for dear life. At last, far down the hall, I saw her surgeon heading our way. I tried to read his body language, his facial expression, then he was opening the door and walking into the room. He came over to us and smiled.

"Everything went well. Lucy is in recovery, and you will be able to see her soon."

We tiptoed into her room. She lay in bed, her eyes closed.

"Lucy. Lucy? It's Dad. Are you awake?" Craig said softly.

She blinked her eyes open. She had a tube down her throat with bandages all around it. She couldn't speak, but once her eyes were open, I could see that she was stunned. One tear rolled slowly down her left cheek, lacerating my heart.

"She's in pain!" I declared. "She needs more medication. She's in pain!"

She looked at me and, almost imperceptibly, nodded.

"Get the nurse! Get the doctor! Help her. Help her! She needs help!" I no longer had any tolerance for watching a child of mine suffer.

"Meem, calm down," Craig said. "Here comes the nurse."

"She needs more pain medication. She's in pain. I know my daughter," I said to the nurse. "She's tough. If she says it hurts, it's seriously bad."

They behaved like I was overreacting, but Lucy's eyes were locked with mine, and I knew I wasn't.

After a few days, they sent her home. She seemed fine, eager to start doing normal things. Her scar was healing in the shape of a little smile just above her collarbone. We went to her postoperative appointments together. She was tranquil, measured. I was in quicksand. The more I moved, the deeper I sank. I couldn't find a tree branch anywhere.

After staying for the surgery, Rose headed out to start a life in New Orleans. Nick continued to shuffle through his existence, not improving but thankfully not deteriorating. I thought I caught some submission in his attitude, a yielding to the illness. The moments when he was present, actually with us, became fewer.

I tried to talk to Lucy about the cancer. Her laconic attitude concerned me. Had there just been so much trauma in this family that we were all turning to stone? Craig and I barely even spoke about Nick anymore. Rose, at nineteen, still held her shoulders constricted, as though trying to loop herself around her pain and contain it.

Brenda's daughter, Lindsay, who had stayed with the girls when we went to France, was getting married. It was the first big outing for Lucy since her surgery, so I took her to buy a new dress. She chose a silvery-beige, backless, sleeveless sheath held together with thin ribbons and tiny bows. We drove out to Malibu for the sunset ceremony. For once, not a single thing was wrong. It felt glorious to be dressed up, celebrating. And together. We sat out on a grassy hillside overlooking the ocean and watched the luminous bride walk down the aisle. She was flushed with excitement and promise. I noticed Lucy, out of the corner of my eye, next to Craig. She sat with impeccable posture, strong shoulders supporting that magnificent head of curling hair. My eyes traveled to her throat. There, just above the Mona Lisa smile of a scar, she'd put two small dots, with a pen, turning it into a happy face.

18

THE WORD

We were on the way home from Beverly Hills. Dr. Amiri had stopped volunteering at the Inglewood Mental Health Center and now saw only private patients. He had continued to see Nick, pro bono. Although I was exceedingly grateful, I now had a constant uneasiness about how long that would last.

"I was wondering, Mom," Nick said.

I prepared myself for some scheme to get me to take him out to eat, or a convoluted math equation that ended with me somehow owing him money.

"Were you, Nicholas?"

"Well, the weekend is coming, and I'd like to relax and watch some TV. I thought, since it was the weekend, you'd support me in getting some Kahlúa, so I could relax."

"All you do is relax," I said.

This was a frequently used tactic. It was either the weekend, or the holiday season, or anytime within two months of his birthday, and that became the reason I should give him extra money.

"Ma, I'm going to really clean up my place today. You know, have a fresh start, so I thought maybe I could get an extra ten dollars." He knew I loved me a good fresh start.

Clearly the Kahlúa was not going to happen.

"I'll tell you what, Nick. How about you come up to the house and you can help me with some gardening? That way you can *earn* some money," I suggested.

"I'll think about it."

After the appointment, he decided he was too tired and needed to go home and rest. He promised he'd walk up later to work. We didn't see him until the next day when he came for dinner.

The day after that he called at 6:30 a.m. "Good morning," he said, cheerful and sounding very normal.

"Nick, I've asked you so many times not to call before eight . . ."

"Guess what?" he continued. "The McRib is back. I thought you might want to go have lunch today."

"How do you even know that?"

"I saw it on a, you know, sign."

"Call me back after eight." This time *I* hung up without saying goodbye.

I hadn't paid much attention to Nick during Lucy's cancer ordeal. I decided he should try the group therapy offered at Kaiser. Since Obamacare launched, Kaiser had restructured its system, and Nick could now return with his Medi-Cal coverage. In the unending, ever-changing labyrinth of a mental health system, I'd almost missed this opportunity.

The first step was an intake appointment. We were meeting with a nurse practitioner who would assess Nick.

"And why is it you are here at the psychiatry department, Nick?"

"Oh, you know, I have some issues with . . . anxiety." His standard reply.

Nick, at twenty-seven, still would not say the word *schizophrenia*. Over the years I'd made sure to vocalize it regularly, for myself as much as for him. In the beginning, he'd cringe, but eventually it was normalized, though he still wouldn't say it.

"Do you have a diagnosis?"

"Well . . . depression and anxiety," Nick replied.

"And what else?" I prompted.

He stared vacantly at the wall.

"Schizophrenia, Nick?"

He flinched slightly, as though touched by a tiny ember.

Walking to the car, he didn't ask to stop for the usual smoke.

"You don't seem to be smoking as much lately," I commented.

"No, I'm not."

"Why do you think that is?"

"It's . . . you know . . . seasonal."

Seasonal.

Two weeks later, we were directed to David Oppenheimer, who led the group therapy meeting. Immediately I felt comfortable. In contrast to the usual bleak rooms with a couple of family photos on the desk, his was covered in original artwork, posters, and memorabilia. I realized, suddenly, that it was the same office they'd taken me to years ago, when Nick had jumped out of the car! Dave Oppenheimer was the counselor who'd calmed me down.

"So, Nick, why are you here?"

"I thought I might join a group meeting."

"Do you have a diagnosis?"

"Schizophrenia." He said the word laboriously, as if it was heavy in his mouth.

And there it was. He had finally said it.

"Well, we have a terrific group that meets on Tuesdays. I'm sure you'll like it."

Nick attended the meetings regularly. The first hurdle, Dave told me, was to get him to take off his sunglasses. That took about four weeks. He rarely participated. When I asked him what they talked about, his response was simple: "Oh, you know—mental health issues."

In late January, Craig went back up to Washington, as was his custom. Lucy decided to move to New Orleans and change her life. She quit her job at Trader Joe's, loaded up her car, and drove across the country to join Rose.

I found myself alone in my big old house for the first time. It echoed with history. I slept in my bedroom, worked in my studio, and occasionally went into the kitchen. How to face those many rooms and what had occurred in them?

I ached for my girls. I wanted them in my arms. I dove into my work, painting like a fiend. Craig was ready to move up to Washington for good; the house was finished, the land cleared and planted. We could move Nick up there near us. But the idea of leaving our house paralyzed me. Every square inch was imbued with the flesh and the soul of my family. I could not imagine releasing this vessel of so much shared history. I created reason after reason why we had to stay. Fabulous jobs, one after the other, anchored me in Los Angeles.

Lucy had settled in New Orleans. She got a job at Delta Air Lines and began to build a life.

Nick continued to attend the group meetings. Kaiser sent email confirmation when he checked in, so I knew he was going. Dave called regularly with updates since Nick had finally signed the HIPAA release. This week Nick had actually spoken, shared an experience. He didn't show up the next week. But after that, he'd not only taken off his sunglasses, he'd participated in a discussion about the challenges of mental illness. Progress.

One afternoon, when I was working in my studio, Nick arrived. The job I was doing involved an interlocking arrangement of stencil designs, requiring math, my nemesis. He stood by.

"Just let me get this part figured out, and then we'll go in the house and get your stuff," I told him. He stared blankly at the desk.

I measured, cut, and tried to fit the pieces together. "Dammit, I don't know what I'm doing wrong."

He walked over to the desk. "Look, Mom." He reached over and picked up the stencil board. "I think this is the problem."

I got up, and he sat down.

"See, if this side is eight inches, then the other one needs to be twelve. That way the curves will line up." He was right.

"Whoa. That's perfect."

"Can we get my stuff now?"

And this is why I can't give up.

I live in a state of constant tension between moments of lucidity and the unknowable. Is he crazy, or isn't he? It's like loving someone who is in a coma but wakes up occasionally to have a conversation with you.

Schizophrenia is bespoke for each person. On the radio, I heard a college professor who had schizophrenia talk about her life. A college professor? How can that be? Why can't *Nick* be a college professor? I am incensed by his foreclosed life.

Nick walked out through Craig's woodshop. He loped toward the house. Our secret garden, cultivated over many years, was green and thriving, even in the dead of winter. The archway Craig had designed to mirror the pitch of the house's roof was covered in white roses.

Nick paused at the back porch to meet Buster. He didn't touch him or greet him, never spoke to him, just stood in quiet communion. He went into the house and a minute later came out with a napkin, flat, on his open palm. On the napkin were two dog biscuits. Buster jumped all around like a screwball but knew to keep a distance until Nick gently placed the napkin into his bowl. A whole bunch of birds alighted on the telephone wires, squawking loudly. We went inside. I made him a sandwich. He took his medicine.

"Thanks for the help with the work, Bub."

"Sure," he said softly as he walked out the door.

I watched his large frame as he headed down the street. It was a cloudy day, and there were no shadows.

I lived alone in the house for a good part of that year. I began taking inventory. It was both a material and metaphysical undertaking. Selling the house was inevitable, and I'd begun, warily, to open closets and look under beds. As I emptied actual boxes, I found myself preoccupied with abstract subjects: existence, losses, truth. I hadn't looked at Nick's writing for a long time. I pledged to read some of it every day. I realized that no one had seen him then or truly known him. Back in the days when he was writing, he was alone in his frightening world. He deserved to be seen, if only in retrospect.

> The music tricks you long term.
> Like my dad's old handwriting,
> which had more of a cursive attribute to it.
> I discovered it on a piece of paper
> in a book I stole from his library.
> fuck!
> I wish I could bring it up to him,
> but he'd concentrate on my crime of theft.

Craig's own father had walked away from his infant son and teenage wife, leaving them to make their own life. Craig had cleaved to his own son with the urgency of the bereft. We all mused that they were like John and Sean Lennon. When schizophrenia scooped Nick up, Craig stood paralyzed as his redemption disappeared in front of his eyes. I ran headlong, haunted and wild, after my son. I am running still.

Rose was not doing well in New Orleans. She and the boyfriend had broken up, and she was couch surfing again. That city was a big petri dish for troubled kids, where their problems would propagate, intermingle with the problems of others, and flourish. Perhaps the heavy, wet air, laden with alcohol, had been the allure. It then became the ruination. Rose wasn't angry with me anymore, and I was grateful for that. But I didn't know how to help her.

"How are you doing, kiddo?"

"Okay, I guess." Her voice was muffled on the phone.

"How is it living with Shannon?" I asked hopefully.

"The place is disgusting. She's got a new boyfriend, so she's never there. It's in a bad neighborhood."

I had asked.

In Lucy's room, I found yearbooks (she'd been the editor), piles of photos, giant-sized birthday cards from her friends. It looked like the typical American childhood. I marveled at the chasm between appearance and substance. I felt like their childhood had been a never-ending sequence of disasters and pain, but everything looked fine in that room. Which was the truth?

"Hey, Lulu, it's Ma."

"Hi, Ma, what's up?"

"Lucy, when you think of your childhood, do you remember it fondly? Were you happy?"

"Of course I was. Why are you asking me this?"

"I don't know. I just feel like the past years have been so awful, like everything is wrecked."

"Mom, you were the best mother. We had the coolest birthday parties, and you cooked really healthy meals every night. We went camping, and you and Dad came to all the school things. We lived in the best neighborhood. My childhood was great. Everyone wanted to be at our house."

That made me feel better momentarily, the images it conjured heartening. But as I sat on her locked storage trunk, I was skeptical. Lucy had moved through the whole experience of having cancer like she was a sleepwalker. She barely spoke about it. I had attributed that to her strength and courage. But what was really going on in there?

That night I lay on my couch with one of Nick's poems.

Are you English?

do you desire overcast deserts?

do you dream of old Italian neighborhoods

in New York?

did you know your grandparents?

did you love to read books?

are you gentle?

are you a fan of the cinema

and solitude in pairs?

television dinners

and apartment plants?

modernist paintings and window blinds?

upstate by acquirement

downtown by chance,

ready for nothing?

Either I was losing all perspective, or Nick's writing was quite good.

When Nick was fifteen, he fell for Emily. She had silken red hair and the olive skin of an Italian maiden. They leaned into each other with the singular trust and abandon of first love. I started to worry about sex.

We were driving to his Boy Scout meeting. "I guess you and Emily are getting serious, huh?"

"Oh God," he said, thrusting as much of his head and torso out the window as humanly possible.

"Nick! You're going to get killed. Sit down!"

He coiled into himself like a fetus.

"I simply want to discuss the issue of you and Emily having a physical relationship."

"Mom!"

"This is the thing . . . I know that the urge to . . ." I faltered.

He was going to cut this off at the pass. "Mom, Emily and I have discussed the question of having sex, and we have decided that we are too young and we want to wait until we are ready, so just drop it."

Hmm. What to make of this? Okay, I'm buyin'. "Well, that is quite responsible and mature of you. I'm happy to hear it."

Of course, they were having sex. Two weeks later I caught him sneaking into the house at one in the morning. I took in the sight before me: my son, sheepishly looking downward, wearing only his boxer shorts.

"Well. Clearly you went out without permission, but the larger issue is this—how could you have left the back door open, to any predator or rapist, with the female contingent of your family vulnerable inside?"

"I didn't want to wake you up opening the door when I got back," he offered.

Good enough.

"Get the hell upstairs, and don't even look at me. I will deal with you tomorrow." My anger, tempered by relief, dissipated quickly.

We never did "deal" with it. Years later, I learned from Emily's mother that they were meeting in the courtyard of Saint Brendan's Church, where they had sex. Why would he bother putting on clothes to go meet her? It made perfect sense.

Some incursions that seemed appalling back then have turned to a different meaning. Now he wanders, alone, down to have a coffee at Peet's. He navigates himself through the tattered souls along Wilshire Boulevard to walk up to our house. Although his days now are barren, I know that he did, at least, have those nights with Emily, the wonder of first love, and I am grateful.

So many things I ignored back then. I just looked the other way because I didn't want it to be true. I wanted our life to be neat like Larchmont Village. These days my cells bang against each other, bruising, and ask, *Did I "let go" of the one thing that might have saved him?*

Those are my stigmata.

"So, what fabulous thing do you have planned for me on Mother's Day, Nick?"

"Hmm. Uh, when is that?" he asked.

"I guess you got it all set up, then?" I said, and waited. "Sunday, Nick. This Sunday."

"Well, can the whole family go out to a nice dinner like we always do?"

"I hate to break it to you, Bub, but you and I *are* the whole family right now."

"Well, how about I take you for a nice meal at Sizzler?"

Mother's Day at Sizzler in a working-class neighborhood of Los Angeles is an experience. We went to Nick's favorite one, sandwiched between Koreatown and a largely Latino area. The entire place was packed with happy families of every persuasion, all dressed up to the nines. Kids ran wild. Several generations occupied each table, the crowning majesty some wizened old lady dressed up like a queen.

At the epicenter of the festivities, Nick and I sat in our usual booth, not speaking. He was pleasant, but when surrounded with pandemonium he turned inward. I was eating ambrosia, seafood salad, and Italian meatballs. Nick kept filling his plate, eating a small amount, and asking for a new plate. A *fresh start*, no doubt. The waitress was not pleased.

"So, Nick, how are you feeling?"

"Fine."

"Are you happy?" Nothing. "Are you sad?"

"No, I'm not," he said slowly.

The answers never changed, but I couldn't stop.

He did say "Happy Mother's Day" as I dropped him off. In honor of the holiday, I went home to do some reading.

I once met a man
Been everywhere in the world.
Matthew Dennis, the man with looks.
He had a brother and a father.
His father died of poverty
and with him stole a son's spirits.
So now his brother eats hamburger.
An artist and a poet,
I love him.
I will never leave him in shame.
Well, we've all sinned,
and I live to forgive.

I saw on Facebook recently that Matthew Dennis is married and just had a baby girl.

Later that evening, Nick texted me: "Hi, it's Nick. Call me back." I called about ten times, but he never answered.

My inventory project moved to Rose's room. I thought of her as a toddler, tough and quiet, Greta Garbo in a backward baseball cap. Nick adored her. Most people thought Rose was standoffish and unfriendly. Nick and I knew she was the funniest thing on two legs. We used to sit in the kitchen and watch her goof around for us; it was a secret we shared. In her night table, I found a photograph of the two of them. Nick was a young boy, holding infant Rose. He is looking at her like she'd just told him the best joke in the world.

In her closet, I found a plastic ziplock bag inside another ziplock bag. *Great*, I thought. *Drugs*. But the bag held the hide of her beloved goat from New Mexico. She had squirreled it away on a top shelf for safekeeping. It was crawling with maggots and growing mold of startling colors. Was there no end to the stomach-turning discoveries my offspring left for me? I ran, holding the bag at arm's length, out to the trash cans.

Nick's entire first year was spent mostly with Craig. I was still working as a scenic artist and was gone for long hours. Craig was working at home, building and painting folding screens, which he sold at a local design store. They spent long days together, Craig working and Nick observing, his ingress into the known world. Nick's favorite lullaby was "Positively 4th Street," sung by his father.

What I remember is the way Craig would carry him as an infant. Nicholas fit perfectly into the crook of his forearm, like a tailor had measured. Craig would walk from room to room, seamlessly, Nick tucked between his wrist and elbow, as though it had been designed that way.

We were at the barbershop again, a grown-ass man and his mother. The thing is, Nick didn't necessarily always seem crazy. He could be well-mannered, quiet. People may have perceived him as mentally challenged, stoned, or maybe having had some sort of head trauma. I doubted that anyone would think *schizophrenia*. After I paid, I'd give him five dollars and he'd go silently tip the stylist himself.

"Nick," I asked, "have you thought about starting to paint again?"

"I'm thinking about it."

"We could go over to Blick after lunch and pick up some supplies."

"I'm kind of tired now, Mom. Maybe later."

"We could just get some pastels."

"I'll think about it."

He's never going to paint again. When I got home, I read some more of his writing, which has the uncanny ability to pull him closer and make him feel farther away at the same time.

> a ferry ride away
> teased dimples and light bangs
> freckles
> laughter

itchy lawn and summer crickets

cold cement front stair walkways

popsicles and shorts

candles and beach haze

tired eyes and feathered comforters

sitcoms and relieving sex

growing old young,

staying young

The few times Nick showed enthusiasm about anything, it involved Craig. In stores, he'd pick up some ridiculous item and say, "Look. I think we should get this for Dad" or "Hey, Dad would like this." At Christmas, Craig was the one person whose gift he cared about.

"Let's get him a thermos."

"A thermos? What does he need that for? He doesn't camp anymore."

We argued, but Nick was emphatic. He picked out a giant one, more than a gallon.

"Seriously? Why so big?"

"For the barn! When he's working in the barn and he wants a cool drink, he won't have to go all the way to the house!" There was nothing I could say—it made sense and showed cognitive activity.

"What color do you think he'd like? Red or blue?" Nick's smile brightened the dismal Rite Aid.

Sometimes Craig would take him out to lunch.

"Mimi, I doubt that he said five words the whole time. He doesn't care."

"That isn't it. He's happy to be with you. It's just sometimes he doesn't talk."

"It's pointless. What is wrong with him?"

"He has schizophrenia. We're lucky he's not just running and screaming through the streets."

"Hey," Craig said, deadpan, "don't confuse me with the facts."

I find comfort in this thought: 1 percent of the population gets schizophrenia. If someone had to get it, maybe it was right that it was Nick who was chosen. I am strong enough to do this. Maybe it was lucky in some roundabout way.

19

SAFE MAGIC

Now that Lucy worked at Delta, Craig and I could fly for free. I wanted—needed—to do some traveling. But I had to figure out a way to leave Nick alone in Los Angeles. A sign of emotional healthiness, or yet another failure as a mother?

This would require outsourcing the duties of administering his medication doses, his apartment cleaning, his laundry. Professionals who make home visits to dispense medication cost a fortune. It's astonishing how many of my friends have done this for me over the years. I have some impressive friends, but I had to find a better solution.

One day it hit me: the halfway house on Crenshaw! That might work. It was just two blocks from Nick's place, and they dispensed medication every day to their *guests*. The place had become even more run-down over the years, but that didn't matter now. He wasn't going to live there.

And so one day I went over to check it out. I walked onto the porch, cement paint peeling everywhere, and knocked on the security screen door.

The man who opened it looked just like Gandalf, long white hair, beard, stooped over—all that was missing was the staff.

"Hi. Excuse me. Is Pearl here?"

"Pearl hasn't worked here in years."

"May I speak with the person in charge?"

"That would be me," Gandalf said.

Gandalf was actually named Roger. He ran the place with the help of Ricky, short for Ricardo. They were a pair, all right. Roger informed me right away that he *used* to have mental illness. Ricky looked like he was straight out of central casting, the hardened ex-con with a lot of tattoos and a heart of gold. I explained why I was there. They didn't seem to think it was weird at all.

"You'll have to talk to Miss Isaac about that," Roger said. "She owns the place."

I called her from the car. She latched on to the "mother" part of the whole thing. She told me she appreciated how hard it must be for me, suggesting we give it a month's try. She'd charge fifty dollars a month.

I brought Nick over to meet Roger and Ricky. As we walked up to the house, we encountered a medium-sized brown dog standing on the sidewalk, alone, right in Nick's path. He and the dog looked at each other.

I waited. "Nick, it's a dog. You can shoo him aside. You're the human."

"It's fine. He'll move soon." His attention returned to the dog. Eventually, I impatiently clapped my hands, and they broke from their reverie.

We were greeted by a friendly guy who introduced himself. It was Robert, the guy who had thought Craig was going to be his roommate so many years ago.

This system we have for the mentally ill is rife with paradoxes. On the one hand, the amount of paperwork required to accomplish anything is ridiculous; the doctors won't even *discuss* your own child without multiple signatures. At the same time, there are board-and-care facilities like this one, where human beings are warehoused, their SSI checks sent directly to the owner. They live in deplorable conditions, and nobody cares. Employees like Roger hand out serious drugs, no signature needed.

I still saw Nick almost every day when I was in LA, but now he didn't call me ten times in a row when he wanted his cigarettes—now, he walked over to Crenshaw. I had not realized the amount of stress our old routine had created until it was gone. I had done it for eight years. Every single day for eight years.

I continued preparing the house for sale. Slowly. I'd know when I was ready. Nick's new arrangement enabled me to spend more time at the farm. Craig was happy.

Lucy seemed good in New Orleans, but I knew Rose was deteriorating. I'd see stuff on Facebook. I'd hear things. She was drinking a lot. I didn't know what to do.

It was June, and I was going to Washington to work on the flower garden. I went to check on things at Nick's before I left. It was in bad shape. I cleaned up, and he took out bags of trash. Alone for a minute in the kitchen, I saw a piece of drawing paper taped on the wall. This was shocking, because he wanted no photos or artwork of any kind. It said, written largely, in his purposeful script:

> After a while what else could I trust but luck
> but truth was the luck.

I was shocked. He hadn't written or drawn anything in ages. The first sentence was in black pencil and the second in red. I didn't say a word about it. I was always barking at him, trying to extract some proof of life. That day I gave him an extra ten bucks without him even asking.

It was beautiful in Washington at that time of year. My dahlias and rhododendrons were blooming, and the sun had returned. I painted, read books, and watched television. Craig was working on his car and installing some light fixtures in the house. I called every day to check on Nick. We were relaxed for once. It stayed that way for about ten days.

About five o'clock on a Sunday morning, which seemed to be the day and time shitty things happened in my life, Lucy called, crying.

"Mom. Mom . . . Rose is in jail."

"Wait. What?" I hadn't had to pull that one out in a while.

"The police took her to jail. I don't know what to doooooooooo . . ." Her voice trailed off like a howling wind.

All I could gather was that Rose had been taken to the local police station in the upper 9th ward. Lucy was hysterical, something about Rose in the back of a squad car, bashing her head against the metal mesh. I told her to calm down and that I'd call her back. With icy calm, I took my laptop into the living room. I was ready to do the thing that I did best: problem solve.

I got on the phone with the local station. She had been taken to central lockup on Dupre Street. They wouldn't tell me anything, said to go to the website. Less than three minutes later, I was staring at my youngest child's mug shot on the computer. She was scowling, eyes defiant. Mount St. Helens gleamed in the background outside our large picture windows. The morning sun was lustrous and clear.

I got back on the telephone and started networking. Craig woke to the happy news. She was charged with resisting arrest, destruction of property, and public intoxication.

Public intoxication? In New Orleans? What, in the name of all that is sacred, does a person have to do to get arrested for *drinking* in New Orleans? For a second, just a quick one, I felt a depraved sense of pride.

I called Jill. She was from New Orleans.

"Rose is in Central Lockup in NOLA," I stated flatly.

"Well, that'll fuck your shit up for a while," she said. "What can I do?"

"Do you know anyone?"

"I'll get back to you." This is a no-questions-asked kind of friend.

By noon she had hooked me up with an attorney who could get things done. I imagine she called in some big favors; she never said. It was what we did for each other.

I got Rose out of jail and on a plane to LA, scheduled to arrive about the same time as Craig and me.

We got there about an hour after Rose's plane landed. By then, supercool problem-solving Mimi had left the building. After endless visions of Rose being shanked in jail, I had dozed for maybe an hour. I woke up thinking I held something in my palm; I could feel the weight of it. It felt like a penknife or a screwdriver. Slowly lifting my arm and opening my hand, I found that it was, of course, nothing.

Once we were off the plane, I ran from the gate down to the luggage area. She was sitting on a bench. Her wan complexion alarmed me. She allowed us to hug her, even reciprocated a bit, but something was wrong. As we walked to the cab, I noticed she was limping.

"What's going on?" I asked, pointing to her left leg.

"Oh, nothing. I cut my knee."

At home I made her take off her pants so I could see. She didn't resist. There was a little tiny cut—like a fish's mouth—white, on her knee. The cut didn't look like much. But the entire knee, out maybe five inches onto her leg in all directions, was a fiery kaleidoscope of crimson. This, I knew, was bad.

"I'm taking her to the emergency room," I told Craig as we flew out the door. No time for questions.

As we drove there, I laid into her. "Rose, I have to say this to you. I know you're sick, and I am most concerned about your health. But I've told you all since you were small that if you ended up in jail not to waste your one call on me. Then it happened, and all I could think of was my nineteen-year-old baby in that terrifying place. But this is it. *You* are paying for the lawyer, and if it ever happens again, I will not pick up the phone. Don't do this to me again, Rose. I cannot take it."

"I'm sorry, Mom."

"I know."

Rose had a serious staph infection. She was immediately admitted and put on strong intravenous antibiotics.

The doctor took out a Sharpie and drew a circle around the red area. "This will tell us if the infection is spreading," he told me in the hall. "I have to say, it's a good thing you brought her in tonight."

Back in her room, I sank into the visitor's chair and once again watched my daughter sleep in a hospital bed.

I woke to Rose's hand on my forearm. "What? Are you okay?" I asked. She did not touch me if she didn't have to.

"Mom, remember a few weeks ago when you sang to me over the phone?"

"Yeah . . ."

"I didn't tell you then, but I'd been wandering around the city, drunk, for hours. Crying. I'd never felt so alone and scared, and then you called." Her doleful green eyes were a mirror. "You stayed on the phone with me the whole time, while I walked home and got into bed. You wouldn't hang up. I was so sad, and then you asked if I wanted you to sing me a lullaby."

The place where her hand had been on my arm was warm, electric.

"Mom, I had been so mean to you, and you just sang me a song. You didn't ask for anything. You just loved me." Her voice, snagged on the words, was breathy and soft. "You just love me. No matter what."

My throat was thick, and I couldn't speak, but I wanted to say *forever . . . always*. I looked at her, my youngest girl, straight at her, and I knew she carried my soul.

My clinging to the house was getting a little ridiculous, even to me, but I saw Nick in every room, and I couldn't let go.

When he was sixteen, he came into his glory. He was handsome, tall, a trendsetter. I saw him sitting at the kitchen table, endlessly drawing, his dark, wavy hair obscuring his face. Leaving to go see the

Rolling Stones with Craig, their arms around each other's shoulders, posing for a photo. He had a beautiful girlfriend—his Emily—who adored him and whom he adored. He had plans. Man, he had plans for his future. Sitting in the window seat, animated, telling me how becoming an Eagle Scout, while not necessarily cool, would help him get into the best colleges. I saw him out on the front balcony, surrounded by his adoring sisters, goofing around. He stood on the porch, leaving for art class, portfolio in hand. How could I ever leave sixteen-year-old Nick?

> I plead forgiveness, acceptance, bliss, ease, purity
> and eternal existence.
> I have an animal instinct
> Let it be forever remembered and breezy like you: delusion or not,
> I beg of you eternity and finesse
> I do not wish to understand my fate
> and endless replenished brain.
> How about unplugging?
> Endless serotonin and ease.
> It will work this time if you grant me this:
> endless energy, mysterious selfness.
> Create the unthinkable and do not look back.

The weight of that single piece of paper unbearable, I let it float to the floor.

I moved on to Rose's room. We were supposed to eliminate clutter and make the house more appealing to buyers, staging it. I boxed things up, marked them *Nick*, *Lucy*, or *Rose*. Finally, the bedroom was back to its original iteration, the perfect little girl's room. As I headed across the hall to Lucy's room, I noticed a piece of a brown paper bag taped above Rose's bookshelf. On it she had written:

And to die is different from
what any one supposed, and luckier.
—*Walt Whitman*

Maybe I was ready to say goodbye to that house after all. I definitely had to get out of there that night.

I went to the local bar, on the ground floor of an old hotel, all by myself. I wanted darkness and anonymity. Of course, I ran into a girl from the neighborhood.

After hellos came the dreaded question, "How is Nick doing?"

"He's all right."

"Can I tell you a story about him?" she asked me. Sour beer smell rose from the metal grate along the bartender's side, and I nodded.

"Remember Nina?" she asked.

Nina had been a tough little tomboy who was in love with Nick when she was seven and he was nine. She grew up to be a steel-strong swan of a girl.

The story took place when the neighborhood girl and the swan were about fifteen years old. They still idolized Nick. One day, he asked them if they'd like to come hang out in his studio. They were thrilled.

They sat surrounded by huge sheets of paper and the detritus of crumbled pastels, crayon, and chalk. Discussing art, politics, and philosophy, they navigated the afternoon. Suddenly, Nick stood up and looked at the swan.

"Wait, don't move," he said.

He walked purposefully across the studio until he was directly in front of the her. He lightly touched her clavicle.

"Do you see? Do you know? Look. What perfect shoulders you have."

Sitting in the inky bar, the girl explained the importance of that moment. It was the first time in her life that she realized a man could appreciate a woman, her beauty, simply for the art of it. Nothing salacious. Nothing sexual. Pure art. She told me it changed the way she saw the world, and men, from that day on.

My crazy son. My insane son. He has changed people's lives.

We put the house on the market in the spring. Rose hadn't returned to New Orleans. City life was destroying her. She had gone up to the farm with Craig to get healthy. I was optimistic.

Over at Crenshaw, Roger and Ricky had been abruptly replaced by Bernadette, an ample, garrulous, Jamaican woman whom I loved. I'd pull into the driveway in my truck, and she'd come out on the back porch.

"Girl, look at you handling that truck. You be just like a man," she'd laugh.

"Gotta be!" I'd call back.

"Aren't you something?"

She took a liking to Nick, and I felt confident she'd look after him. The place was falling apart, but Bernadette brought light with her.

It was Mother's Day again. I drove to the cemetery to sit with my mother. The rituals we move through often bring contentment and meaning, but sometimes they seem artificial. That was one of those times. I went to pick up Nick for—where else?—Sizzler. Our place. On the way we stopped at Crenshaw to drop off his meds.

"Happy Mother's Day, Bernadette," I said. "You're a mother, right?"

"Chile, I have six children. I had seven, but one boy died."

"Oh, I'm so sorry."

"We all have our sorrows," my friend declared. "You and me both."

"So then we'll hold each other up. You and me. And all the mothers."

"That how we stay," Bernadette said.

Nick was in his ninth year since the diagnosis. It was now 2014. I had read, early on, that 25 percent of people with schizophrenia recovered after ten years. It was clear now that he wasn't in that group. I realized that somewhere, deep down, I had been counting on it. Twenty-five percent was a large section of the pie chart. Why not Nick? The possibility had been resting like wings folded tightly against his back all these years, waiting. It was time to admit there would be no flight.

And just to make sure I lost all hope, a notice came from the SSI office. It was time for a "recertification" of Nick's status. They reviewed permanent disability cases periodically to check for fraud. So in case I wasn't sure, I had three weeks of filling out forms, going to the Social Security Administration, and meeting with doctors to reinforce in my own mind that yes, indeed, my son was still, officially, red folder and rubber-stamped insane.

It was time to restock at Crenshaw. I spent the night filling plastic bags like making a recipe I knew by heart: 1 pack cigarettes, 1 ten-dollar bill, 2 Zyprexa, 2 lithium, 1 Strattera. The printed sheet with all his contact and emergency information. This was my ritual, the process of sitting and counting the pills, putting them into little baggies and tying them into little knots. Counting. The days, the money, the pills, the cigarettes—will this be the emblem of my life, this sad routine? I'll never be free of it. And when I am gone, I'll count from the grave.

In the car the next day, Nick began to chuckle.

"What's funny?"

He shook his head.

I asked repeatedly, like knocking on a door. "Nick! You are laughing. It has to be for a reason. WHAT IS FUNNY?" My voice went up into the high registers.

Finally: "Because I am . . ." he paused and strained for the word "happy." It was said not with the conviction of truth, but the relief of remembering the right answer. I stopped harassing him and shut up.

Pulling up at Crenshaw, we were met by several people wandering around outside, smoking. One woman was lying on the lawn.

I took a deep breath. As we walked up the path, a guy said, "Hey, Nick. You got a smoke?"

He nodded and opened his pack to shake one forward so he wouldn't have to touch the guy's hand. Two cigarettes slipped out, and the guy said, "Can I have both?"

"Sure," Nick said.

Inside, I smiled and said a cheery hello to each person we passed. Most were in a daze, but once in a while someone said hello back. I felt an obligation to acknowledge everyone. We got to leave that place; they had to stay.

"Well, there they are! The mama and son," Bernadette said, her syrupy voice a balm. I wanted to lie down in it.

As we walked out, I said to Nick, "This isn't such a bad place, is it?"

"Nah."

"Would you ever want to live in a place like this?"

"No. I like my place, but this must have been a really nice house . . ." He struggled for the expression he was looking for.

"In its day," we both said simultaneously.

Of all the family, only Nick and I are left-handed. One would think that about half the people would be left-handed, but only 10 percent are. I dive repeatedly into the ocean of genetics looking for clues and return empty-handed, left and right.

Spring comes late in Washington; bone-cold tree branches still etched the sky. Southern California was already flourishing—it was always flourishing.

The ten-year mark of Nick's diagnosis was approaching rapidly. I had to accept it. All I had learned through the years—from yoga, from meditating, from having a son with schizophrenia—started to evaporate. I pondered the legacy of hearing voices, being guided by voices. Nick's voices, my voices.

That night it continued to dog me.

I dialed the phone. "Craig, you up?"

"Yeah."

"You know how most people with schizophrenia hear voices?"

"Yes."

"And how almost all of the time they have a similar theme? They are being contacted by aliens or spoken to by God, through the TV, the tinfoil hats?"

"Yeah . . ."

"What if it's real? I mean, what if they *have* been chosen to hear the voice of God? What if they are special, and *we* are the plebeians, the ones who can't tune in to the higher frequencies? In ancient times people with mental illness were revered as holy. What about Joan of Arc? What if, in the grand scheme of things, it turns out that Nick *was* the chosen one? The one who tried to bring us astounding wisdom, but we were too mired in convention to recognize it?"

"It could be," my husband whispered.

"I hope it is," I said. "It fucking better be."

> pleads for forgiveness
>
> wishes to settle
>
> tired of words
>
> wishes for safe magic
>
> the magic that is there
>
> and could learn to grow strong
>
> doesn't mind opinion
>
> wishes companionship
>
> safe desire, afterlife

We sold the house, and I let go. At least I thought I did. We filled up a huge truck and said our farewells. It was late in the evening. I walked through one last time, carefully taking pictures of each room empty. The transformation that occurs when everything is gone is unfortunate. Dirty, sad walls, dotted with clean rectangles where pictures had hung, stare back at you. I thought I saw three-year-old Lucy scoot around a corner, but it was a trick of the eye. The hundred-year-old oak floors gleamed, illuminating the space. I kissed my palm, held it on the front door, and then shut it for the last time.

We had planned to bring Nick up to Washington then, but the behemoth undertaking of just moving us was all we could handle. He was well settled in his routine, and we decided to wait awhile. A friend let me convert her attic into a little atelier, and I came one week a month to fill his prescriptions and spend time with him.

He seemed to be doing well. He looked healthy. He'd lost the extra weight he'd put on when he first started medication. My friends in the neighborhood would see him having a coffee on Larchmont, stop and chat, and report back to me.

Sometimes, in the middle of my day, I'd get a picture on my phone. Nick smiling with a hand up, waving, sent by Jill. Rose had returned to LA after her time in Washington and saw him often. Nothing much really changed in Nick's daily routine.

There was growing evidence that I hadn't exactly let go of the house. When I was in Los Angeles, I found myself driving down our old street every time I could. I told myself it was the fastest route to Nick's.

The first time I actually stopped, it was under the guise of saying hello to the neighbors. I went up and rang their doorbell. No one was home. I stood on the railing of their front porch and peered over the construction fence to see what was going on at my place.

A week later I did see my other neighbor, Amy. I slammed on the brakes.

"Hi, Amy," I said, running up her walkway.

"Oh, Mimi, how are you? How do you like it in Washington?"

"It's great," I said, looking past her at the side of my house. "Have they been doing much work over there?"

"No, they started out like gangbusters, but it seems to have ground to a halt."

"Hmm, looks like the gate is open . . . maybe I'll just have a look."

"I don't know if you're supposed to do that."

I carefully slid in through the semi-open gate. I ambled around, checking things out. It was no big deal.

What started innocently soon devolved into full-on house-stalking.

The next visit to LA, workers had resumed their efforts. I went right on in and introduced myself to Manuel and the guys. I told them who I was, and they gave me the grand tour. It was such an eerie thing, seeing lath and plaster, then naked posts and beams. Like an autopsy. I came back on the weekend and took videos. At this point I was climbing through rubble.

Oh my God, they ripped out the whole kids' bathroom! The hallowed site of my communion with Rose. *How could they?*

Our bathroom was gone too. Completely gone.

Back up in Washington I begged Craig to look at the pictures, to see what was going on.

"Nope. I want to remember it the way it was," he said firmly. "It would just upset me. But, as long as you are now certifiably insane," he added, "the next time you are there trespassing, would you get my vintage *Beware of Dog* sign off the side gate? I forgot to take it."

Well, now I was just acting at the request of my husband. The next time, I cased the joint. The sign was still up, but the gate had been taken off its hinges and was leaning against the house. I returned on Sunday with a few tools slipped into my pockets. I slithered up the driveway only to find that Craig had used the security kind of screws to attach the sign, ones that could not be removed with standard screwdrivers—because we all know about the bands of marauding vintage-dog-sign thieves that roam the city. I tried to pry it off. I tried digging the screws out from behind. Nothing worked.

Before I knew it, I was ripping the wooden gate to pieces with my bare hands, kicking it apart until I had the piece to which the small metal sign was affixed. My mission had gone from covert to wildly, shamelessly public. I sauntered back to my car and threw the huge piece of wood in the back seat. Amy was on her front porch, watching me, shaking her head.

I am ashamed to report that this behavior continued for months, right until the developers who had bought the house put it back on the market. I may or may not have stolen a set of blueprints, which may or may not be squirreled away in Washington. Once I broke in on a weekend and went down into the basement to see how they had dealt with the exaggerated "foundation problems" that had caused two earlier sales to fall apart. I went combat style, elbow dragging myself on my stomach in the crawl space, madly snapping photos of the cripple walls on my phone. Those bastards! Craig had been right; they didn't need to "redo" the foundation!

As I emerged, dusting God knows what off my clothes and hair, Amy had apparently decided it was time for an intervention.

"Mimi, do you really think this is healthy for you? Maybe it is time to let go."

"I know I'm acting nuts, Amy. I do. But I think I'm almost done."

It seemed like she wanted to hug me, but a large moth was furiously trying to escape from my hair, and a puff of dirt floated off of me every time I moved. We just stood there, until I finally said, "Bye, now."

I wasn't even particularly upset or sad during all of this. I was just obsessed. I had a need to watch the destruction and transformation step-by-step, with my own eyes, in order to absorb and to finally accept it. When the remodel was complete and the house was unrecognizable, I let go.

I was in Washington. Having some space between Nick and me was good. I was trying to reignite my own spark and imagine that I could have some kind of a life myself. The concept that I would never be done taking care of him was not an abstraction; it was a fact. I wish I could say, virtuously, that that was fine with me. I'd like to refer to my own musings about *the mothers* and what we do. But after ten years of this shit, I was plain worn out.

I started a bunch of new paintings, working at night and sleeping in the mornings. One was of Lucy sleeping in a meteor shower, painstakingly rendered rocks, iridescent, descending from the sky. I did one of Rose sitting in the yard in LA, her exquisitely muscled arm raised in a plume, covered in a raft of staples from surgery. I painted a self-portrait, my forehead torn after my surgery, with an anonymous hand stroking me gently.

I called Nick one night, late, and he didn't answer. I sat for a while and looked at the dark view.

Craig had gone to sleep. I tried a few more times. The familiar, unwanted nervousness began. I tried to watch a show on television, falling asleep just as it became light out.

When I awoke at noon, I called him. No answer. I called Bernadette. She said he hadn't been over yet. I called him several more times over several hours. I was slipping into the old familiar syndrome, frenzied and certain he was dead.

I couldn't call Rose. She refused to participate in these bouts of anxiety. She said it always turned out to be nothing. And it usually did. But *I* was the one who had been there for the blood, the mouth foaming with pills, the black eyes, and the holes in the wall. I'd patched up the cut wrist. I'd shielded everyone from those things. I sat alone under the weight of a danger proven by things only my eyes had seen. I called my oldest friend; we'd known each other since childhood.

"Hey, Lavina, it's me."

"Hey! What's up?" she answered cheerily.

I explained the situation.

"LJ, I'm so sorry to ask, but could you go over there and check on him? I know he's probably fine, but I'm freaking out up here." I hated myself at that moment.

Rose had the keys, so I told Lavina to just hang for a minute when she arrived at his complex—people went in and out of the locked front door frequently, and she'd be able to sneak in.

For twenty minutes I paced around, sitting down, getting up, scolding myself. The phone, set on silent, vibrated in my hand like a grenade going off. Lavina was at his place. She had gotten into the lobby, but he didn't answer his door. She called him to see if she could hear a ring from inside, but there was nothing.

"Lavina, I think you better call 911," I said quietly but urgently.

The firemen arrived quickly. She explained the situation, making sure that they understood mental illness was a factor. The firemen went in to find the apartment unoccupied. Nosy neighbors milled around.

"What do you want me to do now?" she asked.

"I don't know. I feel like an idiot. I guess you should leave."

I looked at my phone and saw that Bernadette was calling.

"Hang on, it's Bernadette. I'll call you back."

"Hello, darling, this is Bernadette. Your handsome son just came to get his supplies. He seems fine."

I realized what had happened. Nick had slept all day. He'd gotten up and wandered over to Crenshaw. His phone was turned off, as it often is. During that time, the entire production with Lavina and the paramedics played itself out. At some point he returned, unaware, and texted me:

"Hi, Mom, it's Nick. Call me back."

That was it. I called Lavina back and gave her the update.

"I want to tell you something. I am never going to do this again. I am never going to put myself, or the people in my life, through these shenanigans again. I'm done," I said.

"Really?" she asked.

"I mean it. I'll do everything I can for Nick, but this is insane. Ninety-nine out of one hundred times it's not anything terrible. He's asleep, or his phone is off. If I miss that one time, and if he dies or does something irrevocable, so be it. I can't live like this anymore."

"Mimi, you do everything. But this kind of stuff only makes you sick. I really think you have to stop."

"I can't keep going through this. I am done." The clutch of worry holding me, keeping me taut, began to ease.

That night I sat in my studio. Quick glints of light rolled across the walls as trucks went by on the highway. Far away, a siren, or maybe an animal, wailed. I tapped my brush against my shoe.

"I am done," I said again.

And I was. I have not gone to the self-perpetuated crazy place since that night.

20

FEET ADHERE TO SOUL

All of my life, I remember footsteps. One of my earliest memories is of dancing with my father, standing on his feet, like little girls do. I remember walking behind him on the beach, stretching to place my feet into the imprints he'd left. I've always loved the sound of my own footsteps going up and down stairs. The alacrity of my pace a measure of hardiness, stamina. The sound of a lone kid, running down the sidewalk when we were all in class. The definite pound of a heavyset woman. The scampering of young children. The sound of my own mother, walking down the hallway, late at night, safe, safe, safe.

As I began my march toward the tenth anniversary of Nick's diagnosis, I had a lot to mull over. The time had come to look back and reflect, calculate what I had learned. Did I understand *anything*? This was just part of the mission. The other, more important thing was to look again to my son, follow his trail—this journey—over again, but do it now like a pilgrimage. It was time to read the rest of his writing. I owed him that. I had to subdue my own demons, once and for all, and get to a place where I was able to stand and look straight at him. Once I could do that, perhaps I could look straight at myself.

All I dream of is to raise a fine-ass son and daughter
who are happy, vital, intelligent, smoke, drink, paint,
surf, fuck, travel, listen to Bob Dylan, read jazz,
hip-hop, have black friends, have resilience,
be successful
use in moderation, lead, never taken advantage of,
compassionate, caring, crying,
supportive and non-alcoholic

When Nick was twelve, he went to Boy Scout camp and returned with an interesting story.

"Ma, something weird happened when I was at camp."

"What, Nickboy? You can tell me." I steeled myself for the worst.

"I went off by myself for a while. I climbed up a hill away from everyone else. I was just sitting there, looking at the view and thinking about all the beautiful places Dad and I have seen."

"You're really lucky to have had those travels with your dad."

"Then I started to feel funny, like a little sick to my stomach. I was alone in the forest, and I started to feel sort of tiny. Like I was part of a thing, a whole universe, that was way bigger than me."

"That's beautiful."

"I know I have always said that I don't believe in God," my twelve-year-old stated. "And I'm not saying I've changed my mind. But now I think there's a possibility I might be wrong."

I was flying to LA after six weeks away. I'd finally made it to India. I'd saved for a long time for a yoga retreat with my teacher, and now with the free tickets from Lucy, Craig and I both decided to go.

I hadn't been away for this length of time since Nick had gotten sick, and the longer I was away from him, the more I imagined him as he had been before his illness. It would start slowly, subtly, like a winter groundswell. Time passed, and I began to animate his personality, embellish his mannerisms. The magical thinking had gotten way out of hand this time. Maybe it was the wonder of India, but what a shock, what a sad electrical event, to return to Los Angeles and lay eyes on him. Unlike my fantasies, he was muted and remote. His eyes didn't sparkle. His grin didn't dazzle.

I thought of the times—flashes—when I believed he was there for a second. It could be a facial expression, a smile that actually reflected what was going on. Once he'd said, out of nowhere, "Remember when Dad went on the NAMI walk with all of us, at the Santa Monica Promenade? That was nice."

When my mother had been in the hospital, dying, the nurse told us to talk to her because there is some scientific evidence that people in comas can hear what is being said around them. I felt very awkward about this. I could manage it when my brother and sister were there. But sitting alone and talking with an unconscious person, well, it just felt stupid.

On the evening of her last birthday, I'd dragged myself out to the hospital because of the occasion, only to find myself alone with her. I had thought my siblings would be there, but they weren't.

Her room was a peachy color, and the curtain around her bed had sailboats on it. The blanket, tucked neatly around her, was beige. A tray of untouched food lay on the bedside table. Did they really bring food to people in comas? Perhaps the smell of roast beef could wake them up?

"Hi, Ma, it's me, Mimi. Can you hear me? I love you. Do you know where you are?" I felt like a complete idiot. There had to be something more profound to say. But I just kept repeating, "Can you hear me?" like a damn parrot.

Eventually, I sat in silence. I thought about hearing her exhale the word "yes" a week before. It had been emphatic, searing. A final lunge into the world of the living. I sat next to my beautiful mother and considered the sailboats on the curtain. I imagined a fisherman. I could see him right in front of me, smiling and holding a fish. A poor snagged fish flopping through air, seeking water, wanting only that familiar warmth. Oh, my beautiful mother.

She never spoke again. She died the next day.

How will I ever be certain she spoke to me? Maybe I imagined it. Maybe I've imagined all the flares I've thought Nick sent up to let us know his whereabouts. I still wonder, cringing, how long my mother lay on her bedroom floor before they found her. Was it minutes? Was it hours? Days?

The day before the ten-year anniversary of Nick's diagnosis, I didn't know what was real anymore. Would I ever have the wisdom to salvage this hot mess of a life and form it into something of clarity? Would I ever find that simple, perfect place that is the center of the potter's wheel?

> The scary thing is that love is premeditated, anticipated,
> obsessive and reflexive.
> Drives you to a headache
> or feeling pathetic for some reason,
> Narrow down choices, not to worry . . .
> feet adhere to soul.

When we were in India, we visited Varanasi, the holy city that pilgrims travel great distances to see. Bathing in the Ganges River is considered a sacred act. It is believed to wash away sins. Our guides warned us that it would not only wash away one's sins but one's entire immune system as well. Better to stay out.

Our guide in Varanasi was a soulful and gentle man named JP. He took us through the crowded markets and winding streets with a soft *pad, pad, pad* of his comfortable leather-soled shoes. He and Craig formed an instant bond; they both teared up the day they said goodbye. It is a strongly spiritual place, Varanasi. Not everybody likes it. It is crowded and dirty, but it is filled with spectacular colors and pungent smells. The occasional cow wanders freely.

The first day there, JP took us to where the stone of the city meets the Ganges River. He explained the ceremonies that were going on and told us about the history. At one point, I said, "I am a regular practitioner of yoga and a meditator. This place has already taken hold of me. I'm trying to understand so many things."

"Ah, because now you are in the last phase of your life," he said candidly and with intuition.

I started to cry, not because I was sad, but because he was right.

That evening we attended the prayer observance, replete with fire, colored lights, and a brilliant array of the endless hues with which people, clothing, and life presented themselves.

As Craig and JP talked, I wandered away from them. Surveying the vista before me, a familiar sensation began: my face heats, the hurricane wash of salt and water gathers. But no, it wasn't that. It wasn't the sadness—it was some kind of joy. A new kind. Quietly, without drawing attention to myself, I slipped into the damn Ganges River. I needed to shed some sins, and it didn't matter anymore if no one saw me.

Dark water churned as I sank into its consoling warmth. I imagined microbes, universes, ancient particles of carbon swimming gently around me, exploring my ear canals, the inside of my nose, my armpits. I floated on my back and read messages in the stars.

At daybreak, we went on a hushed, solemn ride on the river with JP and two young boys who managed the boat. One of them—a scrappy, clever little guy—was in charge. He watched out for the other, who was bigger and seemed to have some kind of mental deficiency. The littler one rowed those oars with a power that defied his size. When he was spent, he quietly handed the job over to his friend, all the time staying close.

JP gave us each a small tin plate with a candle on it and the petals of a red flower.

He told us that it was tradition to make one important prayer, light the candle, and set it adrift in the river with the petals. I was alone on that boat. Everyone else existed in some other place, far away, as the river flowed by. I put the petals around the candle, hid a few of them in my pocket, lit the candle, and bowed my head.

"It is you," I said to the flame.

As I placed it in the water, I could see tiny lights aglow everywhere. My candle shone like the sun, spinning the world on the tip of its flame. I resolved not to take my eyes off it. At first it was easy, but as the tin plate floated out to merge with so many others, it became more difficult. But I could still find mine—Nicholas. The swishing of the river seemed to emit a clarion call. My promise was that I would keep my eye exactly on him until I no longer could. It began to hurt, this targeted vision, but I held it as the candle faded farther and farther away from me.

"I will watch you. I will always see you," I whispered. Finally, the candle blended into all the others. "Even when I am gone, I will still be here."

It was kind of crazy, I knew, but it was very real as well. It was a promise.

I don't need your genetics anymore.
You might find this hard to believe, but I am very strong.

"Nick, it's your Dad. I know you. You're sharp.
You will be safer, I will change it."

Thanks.

"Yes, you are beautiful.

You're the smartest boy. You'll stay smart. Promise me you'll
beat it.
Shhhh, you there?"

Yep. Crying.

"Please don't listen to their voices.
Remember my smile, I'm your Dadda."

Yeah. Please help me.

"I'm gonna. It'll be good."

Nick wrote that when he was eighteen, alone in his own sea of strangers as his mind turned on him.

It was time to commemorate the anniversary no one was aware of but me: the ten-year mark. The night before, I read a lot of pages in his notebook. With seismic tossing of arms and legs, I remained awake, waiting to find some sort of revelation in the winter of that night. It never came. The day arrived unfettered by my needs.

I'd purposefully taken him out to eat the day before. There would be no commemoration of this anniversary. I only hoped to pass through it with Nick in the world beside me.

"I am not angry anymore," I told the day.

All around me I saw shadows, and in those shadows I saw the mothers.

You hide it in the dark, and it festers and gets worse, I told them. *We need the sun. We need the light of day. We need all the trash piled up on the front porch for the whole neighborhood to see. And we need not to care one whit.*

He has been crazy for one-third of his life. What is it parents always say? *We just want our kids to be content and to be good people.* If that is what we say, then we have to be true to it. I'd be hard put to find a human on the earth who is more intrinsically good than Nicholas Dylan O'Rourke.

The issue of contentedness continues to run serpentine through my soul.

I picked him up, and he said good morning. We went to buy paper towels. We got a few groceries. I took his laundry. We didn't talk much. I went in to see Bernadette while he smoked with the guys outside.

"How you doing, Mama?" she asked.

"Oh, just another day, Bernadette."

I took note of Nick's footsteps as we walked to the car. They weren't decisive. They weren't unshakable. But they did have a confidence about them. He *was* navigating his way. Perhaps Nick had fashioned his own boot-shaped life.

It might be terrible, or it might be just fine.

"See you tomorrow," I told him when I dropped him off at his apartment.

Just let him be who he is. Accept it, I told myself.

After washing his clothes, I sat in my attic, carefully mending some rips. I fashioned precise rows of tiny stitches, ten at a time, tying a small knot at the end of each section. Every time I made a knot, I felt relief.

It was late and quiet by the time I began folding his shirts. I thought that maybe I could hear the sound of ocean meeting the sand, miles away.

> I want lust.
> And then
> not to have to explain myself.
> And then, madness,
> substance,
> breath.

21

THE DUMPSTER

There was a story on the radio about a woman who sells poetry on the street. She sets up a manual typewriter at the farmer's market and sells poems for ten dollars each.

Every time I heard about something that might help explain things, I pursued it. I couldn't leave any stone unturned. The procedure was to tell the poet what you wanted it to be about in a few words. She would take it from there.

"I have an adult son with schizophrenia. I don't know what to do."

She sat for a minute and then haltingly tapped out her verse. It was on a small piece of yellowed paper. She signed it and handed it to me. Holding it in my hand, I walked to the edge of the market and crouched down against a dirty wall. I took a deep breath and then looked at it.

She wrote about time, the undeniability of truth, and humility.

Walking to my car, among carts piled with heads of lettuce and bouquets of multicolored radishes, I read it a few more times. I stopped in front of a table laden with every type of potato in the world and slipped the poem into my pocket. Bouquets of flowers, abundant and bright, lined the sidewalks.

I had moved the furniture from my studio to my little atelier. On top of a beautifully carved sideboard, given to me by Brooke, rest some of my most precious things. I have a collection of painted eggs from all around the world. There is the miniature electric carousel that Lucy and Rose bought me one Christmas. Tiny pins of intricate birds, to put on a lapel, rest in a dish shaped like a leaf. In an arc over the shelf is a string of lights that are fashioned after bright-orange peonies.

At the very center of the shelf is my most treasured possession, my mother's Tibetan prayer box. It is made out of beautiful hand-painted metal and features a little window. It looks like a temple. When you slide the back open, you find another tiny box, an exact replica. My most important mementos reside inside the big box: Clippings of my children's curls from their first haircuts, and their baby teeth. The tassel from the prayer shawl my father was buried in. Dried-up tangerine peels from the day I was brought into my meditation practice. The flower petals from the candle in India. My mother's Red Cross pin. Inside the tiny replica box is a small piece of paper, upon which I wrote the words "His soul is perfect" and folded it in half, twice.

When I returned from the farmer's market, I put the poem into the prayer box.

We decided it was now at last time to bring Nick to Washington. Rose had moved up there with her new, wonderful boyfriend, Aaron, and Nick couldn't stay alone in Los Angeles.

Craig and I created a plan worthy of a military endeavor. In the weeks before Nick's arrival, we set up his new apartment. It was move-in ready. I would fly down, spend a few days and pack him up, then put him on a plane to Seattle. We felt he was stable enough to make the flight alone by then. Craig would meet him at the gate, bring him to his new place, and get him settled. I'd stay in LA for a few more days to empty out the apartment.

At Nick's, I found that most of what was in his large closet was trash—actual trash. Dozens and dozens of the plastic wrapping from his huge paper towel packages. Paper bags. Cardboard boxes. He took all of it to the dumpster. What remained were a couple of big plastic storage containers and a lot of unused linens and cleaning supplies. Carefully placed on a shelf, I found three items that surprised me. Next to his vintage bowling ball (in its bag) sat the bowling shoes Craig had given him on his fifteenth birthday. Next to the shoes was an old plastic train that he'd played with as a toddler at my mother's house. I didn't know he even had that.

"Why do you have that train from Amah's, Nick?"

"You know. Amah."

We argued about which clothes he'd take. I wanted to dispose of them all and get a *fresh start*, but he insisted on taking a few. I allowed those in good condition to be packed in the suitcase.

Before we zipped it shut, Nick placed the plastic train and the bowling shoes on top. He was adamant about bringing the bowling ball as his carry-on item.

"Nick, I was thinking, wouldn't it be nice if you could see a few of your friends before you leave?"

"Sure."

I called Jack, he texted a few friends, and we planned a get-together at Peet's for the afternoon before Nick left.

The next day we went over to Crenshaw to pick up what was left of Nick's meds and say goodbye to Bernadette. The disheveled old place now sat between two brand-new condo buildings, like a crack in a wall. Robert was on the front step.

"Hey, Robert."

"Hello, Mrs. Nick."

I walked around to the back door, where Bernadette was undoubtedly in the kitchen. I gave the screen a knock.

"Hey, girl," she said. "So, this is it?"

"Yep. I'm putting him on a plane the day after tomorrow."

I entered the clean but disorganized kitchen. She handed me his things.

Bernadette took my two shoulders in her soft, weathered hands. "Your son has good manners, and he is strong. I see in his eyes that he is like you. You have done your job, Mama."

I nodded my head slowly, feeling a twinge at the back of my neck, right at the place where there are dead people's bones.

"He is a fine man. That is how he stay." She took me into her arms, and we hugged each other for a long moment. I slipped a Target gift card into her pocket. We said goodbye.

"So I'll pick you up at three, we'll go to Peet's, and then to Danny's for dinner," I told Nick in the car.

At two thirty he called.

"I'm feeling kind of tired, and I thought I'd just rest until we go to dinner."

"Nick! You can't do that. All your friends are coming. I can't reach everyone now. They are all expecting to see you! This is really important." How did I not realize that each sentence was another nail in the coffin?

"Don't overreact, Mom. I'm just going to rest."

He hadn't asked for a party. I had orchestrated the whole thing to prove some kind of a point for myself.

All of it had been my brittle attempt at recreating the past. Instantly, what passed through my mind was the photograph I had envisioned taking. My wonderful son, surrounded by all his friends, the artifact of a fantasy.

All the kids met at Peet's and had a reunion without Nick.

When I picked him up later to go to my brother's, he was a zombie.

At the dinner table, my sister-in-law said, "I don't understand why you don't just let him live with you." My brother glared at her. Suddenly, Nick slammed his hand on the table for no discernable reason. We all flinched. Looking around, I realized—they don't understand. The fear is commensurate with the love. I can't live with him.

Somehow, we made it through the night. I prattled on, trying to fill the awful gaps with small talk. Nick sweated profusely. He made noises. My niece excused herself and went to her room. I did a lot of shrugging.

Finally, it was appropriate to leave. We said some sad-ass perfunctory goodbyes, still trying to feign normalcy. I peeled away from my brother's house like a Band-Aid releasing its wound. I hadn't even reached the freeway when my phone rang.

"Are you okay?" Danny asked me.

I sighed. "It is what it is, and sometimes this is what it is."

"Wow. I'd forgotten. Or maybe I've never seen him like this."

"Yeah," I said, "you'll be walking sideways for a week. Welcome to my world."

"I love you," he said.

"I love you too, DB."

Driving back to Nick's apartment through the expansive hills of the San Fernando Valley, I was soothed by the even geography around me. At my side sat my son's body, but he wasn't there. I had no hypothesis as to where in this world or perhaps some other world he'd gone. My brother and his family were shaken. The Nick they had just witnessed was so far from the boy they remembered and adored. There was nothing anybody could do but take in the natural grace of the planet and hope for the best.

On either side of the freeway, jagged hills held up the night sky.

The last day arrived.

"So, you have your bag all packed and ready. All you need to do in the morning is put your toiletries in and you're good to go. You have your driver's license and Kaiser card in a safe place?"

"No. You threw them away, remember?"

"What?"

"Yeah, when you brushed all the cigarette butts and stuff from my night table into the trash this morning. They were under them."

I abruptly pulled the car to the side of the road. Nick just sat there. I leaned forward and rested my head on the steering wheel. I could feel the topography of my skull, only skin-covered bone to hide and protect the mystery of the brain beneath.

Outside, the traffic rushed up and down La Cienega Boulevard. It was a nice part of town, populated by fashionable people in fancy cars. Maple trees lined the street. At that time of day, the dappled light was like stars. A young woman with a stroller walked by. She was looking at the trees. The small curve of her mouth, her face content and serene. She was wearing slip-on sandals. Short hair and one of those very young, very fresh faces. Unmarked. Because nothing bad had happened to her yet. I could see a little baby foot waving from under the blanket. A bunch of small birds, maybe finches, emerged from the trees and fluttered away, their motion flickering like the dissolution of somebody's dreams.

"Nick! Why didn't you say anything?" I howled.

He shrugged.

"Shrug? You're shrugging? It's a shrug?" I was going downhill fast.

"You were cleaning up," he said.

"Nick," I cried, "this is the post-9/11 world! What are you thinking?" I'm pretty sure he was thinking "What the hell does that even mean?" as I was always saying that to him.

"I'm not going to drive," he said. "I don't drive anymore."

"*That* isn't the problem. They are not going to let you into the airport without identification."

What are we going to do? What are we going to do? My mind was racing. It was two thirty by then. The DMV! We had to rush over there and get some sort of duplicate.

"We're going to the DMV," I announced.

"Can we stop by Old Navy first?"

"Do. Not. Talk." I drove like a maniac.

After the requisite long wait, we were informed that Nick's license had expired. He could get a new one right away, but it would be a temporary.

"Will it have his picture on it?"

Yes. It would be black and white, but it would have a photograph. Nick was going to have to take the written exam. I figured I'd just sidle over and help him a little. We waited in the pool of people for our electronic number to flash.

"You'll have to take off the hat, sir," the disinterested photographer girl instructed Nick as he stood at the counter.

"And the sunglasses."

"For Christ's sake, Nick," I muttered from the chairs.

That done, we headed over to the test line. I coached him up a little.

"Just do the best you can. I'll be over on the side."

As it turned out, the test takers had to go into a separate room with a proctor. No mothers allowed.

"Oh. I can't do that." He said it with a resolve I knew I'd never penetrate.

"Is he going to go in or not?" the clerk snapped. "We can't wait all day, you know. We close at five o'clock."

"You know what?" I asked the clerk as Nick wandered off and dashed hopes bounced all around me.

"Hmm?" she answered, disinterested.

"I hope that one day when you are in trouble, or scared, and the person you are dealing with holds your fate in their hands, that others show you kindness and compassion."

She didn't even look up.

"Well, we're just going to have to find it in the trash," I said decisively.

By then, it was almost five o'clock. Nick was spent. I looked over at the drowsy man-child next to me and knew that, once again, I was on my own. At his apartment he stretched out on the bed.

"Do you remember which dumpster you put the bag in?" I asked preposterously.

He'd already fallen asleep. I looked at his chiseled profile and, hesitantly, reached my hand toward him. I hadn't touched him in years. My index finger reached his earlobe. It was as soft as it had been when he was a baby. I turned my hand and laid the back, not the palm, against his cheek. They say we are all billion-year-old carbon. The side of my boy's face felt as new, as promising, as the day he was born.

The flight departed at seven the next morning. I was wearing a sleeveless shirt, cotton pants, and flip-flops. It was still about eighty degrees outside. I'd ripped my last pair of yellow gloves off my hands in a waterfall of sweat and shoved them into a trash bag earlier that day.

The area behind the building had piles of refuse, old furniture, and broken toys. At the center were two huge industrial-sized dumpsters. I timidly lifted the cover of one. The smell was a mélange of food, urine, and cleaning fluids. Inside lay scores of medium-sized white trash bags exactly like Nick's. It could be any of them. I lifted one up, peering at it to see if I could tell whether it was ours. I tore it open a bit, guardedly, just enough to see tortillas, beer cans, and a big bottle Mountain Dew. Nope.

This went on for a while. Several of the tenants came out, disposing of their own trash. Some looked at me quizzically, while others, recognizing whose mother I was, looked at me with knowing pity. It was difficult to reach into the dumpster; the sides were about five feet high. A beat-up ladder leaned against the building. I dragged it over and continued my search.

The main difficulty was keeping track of what I had looked at and what I hadn't. I started heaving the rejected bags onto the cement. I found a small enclave of Nick bags. Excitedly, I rifled through them. This had to be it! Nope—no license, no Kaiser card, no nothing. Soon I couldn't reach the bags; they were too deep down there.

I stood for a minute in the shade and just stared at the orange sky.

Hoisting myself up, I jumped into the dumpster. It felt like I had landed in hell. It was dark in there. Barehanded, I began sorting through rotten food, used diapers, dirt, bugs, daily household refuse, and squirts and seepages of all kinds amid shards of glass and reeking organic matter.

It was 7:45 p.m. At least it had cooled off a bit. I had been through both dumpsters. I'd found more of Nick's bags, but no license. I couldn't accept that I'd done this unthinkable thing all for nothing. It had to be in there. So I went through everything again.

I never found it.

I awoke before it was light. Looking out the window, I actually got to see the streetlights turn off. I love when that happens. The black sky rolled to indigo and slowly became a washy gray. I'd decided to put my trust in the universe and just go to the airport. Somehow, I was going to convince them to let him through security.

Nick was ready, standing out front with his suitcase and his bowling ball, a big smile on his face. He was excited. I was a nervous wreck.

"This is the deal. I am going to have to convince them to let you in with no ID. You just stand by, don't say anything, and let me handle it."

The first TSA agent we dealt with was a young woman. She had a no-nonsense attitude and basically said we could forget it. He wasn't getting in.

"I truly understand, and respect your authority, but is there by any chance somebody who might be able to make an exception?"

"Well, I can call my supervisor, but he's gonna tell you the same thing," she said.

The supervisor, even more serious, looked at the papers I had tried to cobble together as some semblance of identification. Craig had sent me a scan of Nick's expired passport and his birth certificate. The supervisor just said no, this nonsense would not do.

Crestfallen, I crouched down and hung my head. All around me, active and engaged travelers moved toward their destinations. They had briefcases, backpacks, spiffy rolling carry-ons—all the things that signified productive lives. Looking up at them from my diminutive position, I was overcome by their success and my inability to just grab my son and join their ranks.

"Would this help?" Nick said, excavating something from deep in his pants pocket.

He handed a card to the agent. It was his Metro card, current, replete with a color photograph and an identification number.

"Oh. This is fine. Go on through," the tough, unyielding TSA guy said.

I jumped to my feet with the agility only an old yogi could muster. I felt I might have hit the ceiling.

"Really, Nick? Really? You couldn't have shown me that before I swam in raw sewage for three hours?" My voice held only irony, no malice. I almost started laughing.

"I didn't know you wanted that," Nick said, gazing off into space. "You could have just asked."

The church that sits kitty-corner to Nick's old building hosts many events. I had seen many fluffy brides and nervous grooms outside. Bleak faces of mourners, gathering to reminisce, milling around the entry. I trusted they all somehow watched over my boy of unsound mind. Between events, the grand steps served as a meeting place for the old women of the neighborhood. They sat with thick nylon stockings rolled above their knees, looking more like big dolls than old ladies. I'd see them snicker when someone walked by or lean together and fervently whisper secrets no one else even wanted to know. They clearly knew everyone's story. I'm sure they knew mine. I had to park right in front of them on my way to clean Nick's place. They clammed up until I crossed the street, and then they all started talking at once.

Inside the walls of that apartment lived the history of my family's worst calamity and the evidence of its most tenacious love. If I could have, I would have set a match to all of it. I would have set the love afire to eliminate any trace of the scourge. All day I carried crap out to the dumpsters. At the back of his closet I found yet another box, with a bunch of notebooks stuffed inside. I dragged it across the grimy floor into the living room, where I opened one. The date read September 2002. It was a journal from the year he'd cut his wrist!

When I realized what I was holding, I slammed it shut and lowered myself down into child's pose. There was a notebook in that room that might explain, in Nick's own hand, what had been going on in his head when it had all begun. Was there some answer within reach?

That box and I were like two giant magnets, repelling and pulling. I kicked the box into a corner and glared at it. It was a typical moving box, brown with dented corners, the word MEDIUM faded across the side.

I picked up a flimsy IKEA cabinet, hoisted it over my head, and retreated down the hall while emitting a dull, guttural growl. The rectangle of light that was the back door seemed a hundred miles away. Once outside, I threw the cabinet against the wall. It broke into several pieces. That wasn't good enough for me. I ripped the drawers apart.

Then I did a thing I'd seen men do but had never understood until that moment. I started kicking and punching the metal dumpster like a maniac. It felt good. I kept going. At the end of it, knuckles bloody and knees scraped, I'd found some kind of crazy comfort.

As I stood there trying to catch my breath, I thought of the holes in Nick's walls. Yes, holes punched in walls are born of anger, but of what is the anger born? I had assumed it was something grotesque, reprobate. A beastly presence bent on destruction. I knew right then, fingers throbbing, that it could be created by something else; it *could* be born of love. All this destruction, the rage, the longing, could come out of love. My love for my son. A terrible love that claws at my insides and makes the idea of punching walls seem soothing, but love nonetheless. Could it be the same for Nick? Is there a path to peace through ruckus?

I returned to the work at hand. I decided to get the bed out. Figuring it was best not to dump *two* vermin-infested mattresses in front of the same church in one lifetime, I knew I had to put it in the dumpster. Not easy. But I returned to the apartment with a slight skip in my step. Feeling rather strong all of a sudden, I read some of the notebook, smearing the blood from my hands onto the pages. When I couldn't take any more, I detonated six insect foggers in the apartment and went to yoga class. Namaste, baby.

Over the course of that week, a feral seed had taken root. I developed an irrational conviction that if, somehow, I could get the majority of the security deposit back, it would be redemption. It would say: *a human being of worth had lived here.* Not an animal. Not a madman. A person. That security deposit would be my proof.

After yoga I went back down there. I began to transform the space into an acceptable condition. I worked late into the night, walking ever so lightly and taking care not to let the metal security screen slam. All the while, the box of Nick's journals jeered at me from the corner of the room.

I returned to my peaceful attic in the early hours of Friday morning with the box. The contrast between the two places was the saddest story ever told. As I sank into the plush comforter on my bed, I marveled at the disparity of lives, of circumstances. There is no order to the universe, only the caprice of nature colliding with the imperfection of humans.

Now that I was intent on getting the deposit back, I went to work with enthusiasm. At the end of it, the apartment looked like new.

There was a bed-sized square of carpet that was clean, still beige. Next to that was a mid-century night table that had been a polished teak once upon a time.

Years before, when we returned from Paris and Nick was setting up his new bedroom in the TV room, we'd gone to a few used furniture shops.

"Hey, Mom, look at that!" He pointed to the curb as we drove home. Sitting on the grass next to someone's trash cans was a small table. It was pretty beat-up and one leg was broken, but it had a lot of style. "I'm going take that, Mom, it's perfect. Do you think it's okay to take it?"

"It's a mess, Nick. You'll have to do a lot of work to get it looking good."

"I know, but it'll be fun. I'm taking it."

That table was Nick's first project in the backyard art studio, back when he was eighteen. He glued the leg back on as his father had taught him to do. He painstakingly sanded the surface with increasingly finer papers to close the grain. He oiled and polished it to a golden finish. Sitting on a clean drop cloth on the green grass, it looked fit for a museum.

The teak table was where Nick now kept his ashtray. The top shelf was completely black from a quarter-inch layer of soot. The second shelf was a sticky layer of old soda and food. Dust, dead insects, and matches stuck to it like some kind of macabre collage.

I started washing it. Initially, I was just curious to see if it was possible to clean something that dirty. After about three go-rounds, I started to see the wood under all the cigarette ash on top. I got fired up. I tried the second shelf. That required steel wool, but it was coming off. I scrubbed the top back to the clean wood surface. It was dry and faded, but was it possible that something so degraded, so ruined, could actually be saved?

I scraped and scoured and removed every bit of dirt from that table. Then I refilled my bucket with clean soapy water and tenderly washed it once more. "There you go," I said out loud. I got a towel and thoroughly dried it. I decided to take it with me.

I stood at the door looking back into the apartment. The empty rooms sat before me like a decrepit theater, exhausted from all the dramas, the comedies, the lines recited again and again. In the way a photograph negative reverses light and dark, the carpet mapped out where there had been furniture.

I returned the keys to the disdainful manager upstairs and left.

22

IN THE SWEET BY AND BY

I was left with a few more days in Los Angeles all to myself. I drove up Norton Avenue one last time. Looking at the now pale-gray, perfect house, I was surprised to see the family sitting on the front porch. People didn't do that in the neighborhood anymore; everyone is much too busy. I slowed down.

Parking under the huge magnolia tree that had provided dappled shade in my life for twenty years, I looked furtively at the house. A new, stylish retaining wall had been built, curving around to contain the constantly crumbling corner of the lawn that we'd just lived with. Several of the outlandish number of trees Craig had planted were gone; there was finally sunlight on the house. A good-looking man and woman sat with two young girls on the steps. A floppy magnolia bloom dropped and rolled leisurely across my windshield, over the hood, and onto the street. I took that as a sign, got out of the car, and walked up to the house.

"Hi, do you live here?"

"Yes," the dad said slowly, cautiously.

"I just wanted to say hello. I'm the person who lived here before you." *This was a stupid idea. What would they care?*

"You're Mimi?" the man said incredulously. *Yikes. What has been said? God help us all if those walls could talk.*

"Yes . . . I'm Mimi."

"Oh, we're so happy to meet you. We've heard so much about you. Everyone on this block *loves* you guys!"

Introductions all around, some small talk, and then there was nothing more to say. The front porch was brand new; they'd rebuilt our old collapsing one. The hibiscus bushes I'd planted still lined the south border of the lawn; their barely sweet scent hung in the air. I looked up at the hidden corner of the porch roof, where Rose used to crouch and hide when she was mad or in trouble. Looking at the flower beds, I could see Nick, about nine, kneeling with Craig on a Saturday morning as they pulled weeds. For some reason, I thought of the time I'd hidden on the porch for forty-five minutes with a raccoon mask on to startle Lucy, who'd told me she'd had a scary dream about a raccoon. We had rolled on the grass, laughing.

I remembered Craig and me, in the driveway, sobbing, the day we admitted to each other that Nick was lost. I saw all the kids playing Ping-Pong in the porte cochere, joking and quarreling. I looked down at my feet, firmly resting on the cement walkway we'd poured ourselves the first year we had lived there.

"I'm really happy to have met you," I said. "It is so good to know that nice people live here. This house will always be in my heart. So. Have a life!" I held both palms up to either side with a shrug.

I haven't driven down Norton Avenue since.

Back at the attic, I decided to do some reading. The loathsome box sat on the floor, beckoning me onto treacherous cliffs. I opened the first notebook. September 2002.

> I crack my knuckles like crimes galore
> knead my palms and
> grease my cheekbones

grease my cheek loans
freak my weak phones.
And fix my pick finger with band-aids and ointments.
I'm like an October fallen leaf
and I'll find my love one day.
Somehow get home
to your sweet smile.

There was a bundle of poems written on the back of some printed matter. After poring over pages of scrawled cries for help, made-up words, and gibberish, I noticed what they were written on—faded printouts from the internet on living with bipolar disorder. Under the section titled "You Are Not Alone," he had marked some words and phrases with a highlighter: *a treatable disease*; *how others have experienced anger*; *alcoholism, drug abuse, and other self-destructive behaviors*; *a chance to lead a normal life.* "I can do this" was written at the bottom, in Nick's cursive, with a yellow highlighter. I carefully folded that one into a paper airplane and sailed it across the room.

His initial notebooks, when the disease was emerging, held neatly penned ideas in complete sentences. As it progressed, the script got sloppier, and he changed colored pencils often. The poems became blatant calls for help. Requests for another chance. Promises of reformation. Then he started writing on anything—art paper, brown bags, napkins. His sentences no longer held level; they curved downward, as if falling off the page. Soon enough, he was writing in every direction, in spiraling circles, upside down. Finally, on the last papers, they weren't even words anymore. There were just letters and punctuation, a language known only to him. A miasma of sorrow was all I could see.

After a while, if you're lucky,
you'll find that as an artist you'll
arrive at a flow that is
your style of painting.

And, sticking to it, you'll develop a sort of font
that can be recognized as
something you've written.

Oh, I had been lost for so long in the mist of thwarted mothering, trying, trying, trying to be something I'm not. I had wanted so badly to put on the costume of the perfect matriarch, dressing the whole damn family up to match. But we never belonged in Larchmont Village. The fact is we were always a couple of outsiders there, Craig and I, as best illustrated by our son: skinny, maniacal, gleaming with a sweat mist of his own, running through the streets of the neighborhood in skull-decorated swimming trunks.

Who did I think we were fooling? We couldn't even fool ourselves.

Dr. Amiri had canceled his last meeting with Nick because of a family emergency. Nick had left the next day. Rod Amiri had been Nick's doctor for ten years and never charged a cent. This man had been the singular redress in a mental health system that had let us down in almost every way. He had been the first doctor to diagnose schizophrenia. I made an appointment to see him myself and say goodbye.

"Mimi, I feel awful about missing my last meeting with Nick."

"It's okay. I explained that it was a family issue, and he understood."

"My mother died that day," he replied in an even voice.

"Oh, I'm so sorry," I sighed.

We proceeded to have a personal conversation for the first time. He told me how close he'd been to his mother. They'd even lived on the same street. He said he wasn't sure how he felt; it was all just sinking in. I told him about my mother dying and that I don't think you ever really "get over" it, you just carry it. It was a strange and galvanizing interaction, the patient's mother consoling the doctor who had just lost his mother.

The night before, I had gone through some of my paintings. I picked one out; it depicts a man in a suit, blowing hundreds of tiny pieces of paper, causing them to swirl around his head. I wrapped the painting in plain brown paper and tied a piece of string around it. At the end of our conversation, I gave Dr. Amiri the painting.

"You saved us," I said before I left his office for the last time. I was overcome and didn't want him to see me cry. I left before he could open it.

At home, I waited to hear about the security deposit on the apartment while reading.

> I plead forgiveness, acceptance,
> bliss, power,
> ease, purity and eternal existence.
> I have an animal instinct
> Let it be forever
> remembered
> and breezy like you,
> delusion or not.
> I beg of you:
> eternity and finesse.
> I do not wish to understand my fate.
> An endless replenished brain,
> How about unplugging?

The muscle that is my heart careened around my chest cavity, bouncing off my rib cage like a pinball, finally tumbling into a dark hole. I couldn't read any more.

I received a message from the management company informing me that I could come by and pick up a check. They had inspected Nick's apartment and an assessment had been made. The original deposit had been $875. I was positive I'd be getting a check for some joke amount like sixty-three cents.

I ripped open the envelope in the office—$875! I had done it. I had taken that godforsaken pit and resurrected it.

Anything was possible.

That last night I read more. A small chandelier that I made myself hangs in my attic. I bought an old fixture at a swap meet and replaced the clear crystals with a dazzling assortment of colored ones. It is the prettiest thing ever. It throws delightful prisms all over the room, which dance around when any wind moves through. I liked to lie on the floor and just stare up at it. That was what I was doing, surrounded by Nick's scribbles and drawings.

> It's interesting to see myself grow into a being
> day by day
> through ups and downs.
> You look back through certain memories
> and you grow stronger.
> You realize how vulnerable the past is,
> every moment recollected and reanalyzed,
> held on to or forgotten.

"This hurts," I told the night. "This hurts my body. Why do I have to read this?"

> I have been so far gone from a man with success and happiness
> that I feel a state of uncertainty as to whether I deserve a recovery.

"Why do I have to know this?" I asked my chandelier.

> I would like to move upstate, Ma dear,
> and I wood like to move upstate. I would like to

plant a tree in my own little yard
and then create a garden.
I wish I had children.

I rolled over onto my belly, resting my forehead on the tops of my hands. "I preferred it when it all was a mystery," I told the rug.

Whah? Yeah?
Send the reminder
that the time has come around in your life,
the time you could remember.
Before and after threat and fear,
when we arrive at the fact that there's
a crack in the ice
and it's quickly tearin'
up in between your feet.

I sat up. I noticed the night table, shoved in the corner of the attic.

And while you're at it
remind me not to have taken note
of the last few years.
When a good idea traps, throughout you,
assumptions that were made, and
the seesaw keeps fucking
slapping back and forth
until, one day,
you'll piss yourself.

"Fuck you," I sneered at the night table.

I could either lay around and
drool, or one day
my heart would catch up
with something.
Christ, some plateau perhaps.
Naked and bleached
by the day cold heat
of morning time,
in a campsite,
next to a reservoir.
railroad tracks
New Morning.

That was the 2002 road trip to Uncle Cal's funeral. The video I'd found of Nick and Craig, laughing. I stood, with an ache in my gut so powerful I felt it in my jaw.

I went over to the table. I ran my palms over the surface. It was rough. The teak was almost white. After all it had been through, it was dry as a bone in the desert no one knew about. The repair Nick did to the leg had held. The jumpy lights from my chandelier could be seen in the window, but the wood was so parched it had no sheen. No reflection was possible there.

"It is not over yet," I told the table with authority.

I returned to reading. For a period of time, all he wrote were lists.

Ninety miles an hour
A variable shelf of silver
Hey, odelay
Denny dentist dental mints floss bowtie dickies satin satin
I like Pink Floyd. And Converse. And change. Ha
Sonic youth. Red. Drumstick. God. Burrito. Theater.

"That's some crazy-ass shit," I told the paper. The last thing I read in my son's journals that night was this:

> Yes, lord, I have sinned a great deal
> and would like to change.
> Can you forgive me?
> Can I hold your fragile mind and mix
> my drink around for a bit?
> The smells are funny and vanilla shoots forward
> and I would like to be alone and sit on this success.

At that moment, I knew what I was going to do.

I wasn't sure when—there was no rush—but I could envision each step of the process in perfect detail. First, I'll get some 180-grit sandpaper for wood and tenderly sand the night table to settle the grain. Next, I'll take a quarter sheet of 220 and smooth it even more. Then, oil it. I'll do it a couple of times. That table is thirsty. After a couple of days drying time, I'll take the softest cotton rag I can find and buff that baby right back to her former glory, quickly and with a light hand. The heat from the gentle friction will make the teak blossom, breathe. One more fresh start.

"Put that in your pipe and smoke it," I told the solemn night.

I had hoped the conclusion of this story would be about some sort of perfect acceptance, a surrender, like they teach in yogic philosophy. But no, messy world, this was not attainable. Instead, I have managed to incorporate Nick's madness, invent a life for us where it can reside. We stand in mountain pose, he and I, palms forward, shadows behind us. Insanity—I will never make friends with its rodent soul. I have learned that even near-perfect acceptance includes movement, discord. I live with the truth that I have met my match but not my conqueror. There will be no surrender. I walk in my own footsteps now, not counterfeit ones, in love with the radiant brightness of it all.

Lying back on the floor of my little attic, I stared out the window to the moonless sky.

As if it were possible to record the actual sound, the smashing upon smashing his recollections made as the deconstruction of his mind proceeded, he had scrawled words and letters on these pages. They were not meant for me, and yet I feel like they are mine, part of him, as he is part of me. I had some hesitation about reading them, but now I believe it is my due. I have earned this intimacy.

My job is to be the conservator of his legacy. Yes, the universe has decreed his fate; there is no mitigation of that edict. Nonetheless, I am going to keep alive the possibility of a better ending. It is, admittedly, a tattered, decomposing rope I hold. But he is there on the other end. My job is to wrap my tough, arthritic knuckles around it and not let go.

I do believe, now certainly, that my mother said "yes" out loud to me in the emergency room. Moving toward her deathbed, she gave me that. It was the last word she uttered on this natural earth. The precise center of the potter's wheel. Every single time I look into Nick's eyes, I will hear that *yes*. Resounding. Definite. Irrefutable.

EPILOGUE

It is the spring of 2017, and two years have passed since Nick moved up to Washington. He lives in a nice apartment now, kept clean with the help of DHS caregivers. He has an attentive doctor and kind neighbors. The support system in Washington is far better than in California. His life has settled into an even rhythm. He watches television, colors in coloring books, takes walks. The lush green and the immaculate air of the Pacific Northwest seem to do him good.

A warm wind blows from the past. I am at the top of a hill overlooking a valley of olive trees in Jerusalem.

Sara needed help after back surgery she'd had done in Israel. Sometimes life serves up exactly what you require. I was caring for my sister and wandering around the place I had feared wasn't real anymore. When I'd left, it was like the final time you make love with somebody; I didn't know it was the last time. The years piled on, and the memories began to seem like dreams. Now they are real again. I visited my old house. Covered with salty mud, I walked into the Dead Sea. I still understand the language, and that was a surprise. Something has been restored inside of me, an important chunk of my life that had slipped into darkness. Nothing is lost. It was only resting, like an indolent hound, waiting to be gently nudged awake and fed.

I cook for her, change the dressing on her incision, and accompany her to doctor's visits. I am grateful for this opportunity, to take care of her, to relive our childhood. Outside the window, city lights shimmer and a baby moon is pinned above us. Not quite a crescent, it is smaller—like a perfect, tapered slice of the best cheese. My phone begins to vibrate, telling me I have texts.

"hey its nick. call me back"

"hey its nick. call me back"

"please call me back"

"why won't you call me?"

"Do you think he wants you to call him?" Sara asks.

"Hi-larious," I say, dialing his number. "Hey, it's Ma. What's up?"

"I want you to send me the phone numbers of my friends. Can you do that? Milton, Jack, Itaru, Jenny, and Chris Collins." He was speaking very fast.

"Why, Nick?"

"Because I want to reconnect. I want to talk to them and say hello."

"Okay, I'll text you the numbers." My voice has the timbre of either excitement or fear; even I don't know which yet.

"So?" Sara asks.

"I don't know. Maybe it's a good thing. Maybe not. He wants to call his old friends. I think it could be good. You know, showing signs of interest in others?"

I send individual texts to Nick with each friend's name and number, so he won't get confused. Falling asleep that night I imagine a fairy tale where he gets better. It all starts when he decides to call his old friends.

A sovereign dawn arrives in Jerusalem, and I am awake to meet it. My sister sleeps in the next room, her body slowly healing. I look at my silenced phone. There are several texts from Nick:

"22 texas holdem"

"cable. licorice. mayo. cardboard. plastic. drywall. matrix. seal trucker."

"Scientology. hookah. aerosol paint. toothpaste. tea. vitamin."

"pb and j. Transylvania. Christ. apple pie. lavish bread. mattress.."

I don't want this. I don't want these messages from him. I just want to be here in this place with my sister and reimagine my youth. What am I supposed to do about my crazy son from across the globe?

Midmorning brilliance fills the room as I make the coffee. Sara wanders in, and I show her the phone.

"here comes Santa"

"I need extracurricular activities. And new shoes. And cable. Bacon."

"Can we go to burning man?"

"Whoa," she whispers, "what is going on?"

"I don't know. This is so shocking. It's like the writing he used to do in his notebooks, way back when he was first going nuts. But he hasn't written anything in years, and he's certainly *never* texted like this."

"What are you going to do?"

I look out the glass at the city before us.

"You know what I am going to do? I am going to make your breakfast, and when you take your nap, I'm going to the Western Wall and the Old City. Fuck it. Maybe this is just a glitch or something. Maybe it will just go away."

My sister gives me a look that only one who understands your terror can summon.

"Sure, no reason to overreact."

By evening, my phone is filled with nonsensical strings of words. I am tripping all over them as I enter the apartment.

After several conversations with Craig and then the girls, a picture emerges. Nick's rambling texts had been boomeranging around the stratosphere, like shrapnel, for the past twenty-four hours. For once, no one wanted to upset me—a reverse of our decade of family dynamics; they had kept the phone messages to themselves.

I am half falling off the child-size futon in my room, my legs contorted in extreme yoga stretches, phone wedged between my neck and my shoulder. "What the hell, Craig? What is this? What do we do?"

"Miriam, it's just more of the crazy. You can't do anything. Take care of Sara, and be in Israel. You are finally there. Just be in the moment. I will take care of Nick."

I decide to listen to him, for a change. The next day I go to the top of Masada, where the last Zealots chose suicide over enslavement. I pay my respects. I eat a falafel. I tend to my sister. I remember what it was like to be seventeen, living in Jerusalem. I wander the white beaches of Tel Aviv by myself and recall the terrible loneliness of adolescence. I eat another falafel. Sara gets better.

After ten days, I head homeward.

On the flight, I take stock. Our lives were decimated for a decade, so where has my family landed? There were years when we were lost to the wind, twisting and slamming against each other relentlessly. Now, Rose and Aaron are married and live happily on their land in the country. Lucy is healthy, in love, and traveling the world. Scarlett and her husband are raising their seven kids in rural Texas. Craig and I perch on our ridgeline overlooking Mount St. Helens, its sheared horizontal crest a reminder that nature does destroy but is dogged in her resilience. We don't live in a big, impressive house anymore. Out my window now, goats wander the untamed property and there a lush, sloppy garden. Suddenly, with a spark of recognition, I see the farm painting Nick did when he seven years old, out in his dad's studio—the cows, the chickens, the gradated blue sky. Here, the sky moves from pale cobalt to ruddy blue-orange into a prescient near black. The sun has just set.

We found our way back to our marriage. We hold the elusive gift that is real love carefully now. Time and struggle have shown us its worth. Our boy still has schizophrenia, and that is never going away. But he is content, peaceful these days. Things could be worse.

I am fearless in front of the mirror now.

Home in Onalaska, it is raining. In the drizzle and the half-light, I drive into town to see him.

"What, Nick? What are all these texts?" I stand in his sparse apartment and try to understand.

"It's poetry, Ma. I'm writing beat poetry again, on AOL!" (AOL?) His face opens into that shock of a grin that stops time.

"Nick. It is great that you are writing poetry. It's fine to send it to Dad and me. To Lucy and Rose. But you can't send this stuff to your landlord. He is not going to understand and will just think you're annoying. You don't want to get evicted." I remove the scarf and shoelaces he has pinned to his front door.

"Why are these here, Nick?"

"You know, for New Year's," he says. My sadness bounces off the fact that it is June.

Suddenly, I have one of those memories, and the sweet idiosyncratic nature of Nick as a small boy becomes telling, prophetic.

When Nick was about four years old, he developed a funny habit. We'd be sitting on the couch, watching TV or just relaxing, and suddenly his attention would be drawn toward and then riveted by some unidentifiable thing across the room. He'd stare for a while before deliberately walking over, bending down, and picking up some minuscule crumb from the floor. Holding it in his small palm, like it was a gem, he'd bring it to me as a gift. A speck. Is that what these texts are? More specks? Perhaps they are jewels, or maybe they are just dust. And then I think, *They are both.*

I have been home for a few weeks now. Nick is exhibiting an astonishing shift in behavior. He continues to text furiously, often late at night. I bought him a large notebook, which he filled with his poetry in two days. He is talkative and engaged with others. Some of the changes are troubling. His landlord reported finding a loaf of bread and a container of hummus in the dryer of the laundry room next to his apartment. He denies any involvement. He gets agitated when trying to convince me to do something. I don't think he's sleeping. He is also on the internet for the first time in years. He made a Facebook page and listed the woman he stalked so long ago as his employer.

I have been visiting all the professionals: the doctors, the social workers, the caretakers. No one knows what the hell is going on.

I even had Nick's astrological chart done by a friend. She calls me the same night and says, "Mimi. He came in with it. Every single signifier and indicator for mental illness, he has it. It was there from the beginning," she says sadly. "He came in with it."

I call Dr. Amiri in Los Angeles.

"I don't know," I say. "This seems like it may not be a bad thing. It's like he's waking up or something."

"I agree, Mimi, but any deviation from an established baseline has to be taken seriously. If you are positive that he is taking his medication, I think he needs to see a psychiatrist to be evaluated. A change like this could also indicate decompensation."

I don't want to ask him what that means because I hate the way it sounds.

The rain is like rocks on the roof. It is the deep of the night. I sit alone at my computer and do a search: *What is decompensation?*

This term describes the worsening of an individual's mental health. This occurs in persons who previously had control of their mental condition. Decompensation results in a decreased capacity to engage in ordinary daily activities, episodes of worsening symptoms of this mental disorder. Patients also exhibit bizarre or violent behavior at times, insomnia, and paranoia.

Well, nothing is mentioned specifically about bread and hummus in the dryer, so I decide this clearly doesn't apply to Nick. I stare at the screen as sophistry takes over.

Yesterday I introduced Nick to a woman I know, and he stepped toward her, held out his hand, and said, "Pleased to meet you." I stood by, speechless.

Before I go to bed that night, I text him:

> "Nick, I love you very much. You are my firstborn and the light of my life. Please always remember this."

I know I won't get a response, but I don't care. The next morning this arrives on my phone:

> "Aw, that's so nice. I was just making my morning coffee and I saw your text!"

Happy, I drive to town and meet him at the art supply store. He rushes up to me, visibly excited. "Mom, come here. You've got to see this!" He brings me to a rack of postcards and points to a large Technicolor image of Mount Rainier. "Look! Isn't that *amazing?*"

He's noticing beauty and wants to share the experience?

The next morning at 3:00 a.m., Craig gets a text:

> "Are we ever going to ever go camping in Sequoia again, this summer, or even hiking?"

Nick is being reevaluated by the social worker because of the changes in his behavior. She asks him if he knows what month it is. He does not. She asks him if he can clip his own toenails. He smiles. She gives him a pad and a pencil and tells him to write a sentence. Any sentence. He stares at her and shakes his head no. She hands him a fairly complicated geometric design and asks him to try and reproduce it as best he can. In about twenty seconds he has drawn a perfect replica. She is stunned. I am not.

Days pass. The morning light lands on our valley, articulating the trees like a fine pencil drawing. I go to his doctor appointments, talk on the phone, write emails. Is this just a random manic episode that will pass, and will he return to normal-crazy? Is he—dare I even say the words—getting better? Or is it the precursor to decompensation? My head spins. No definite answers. Never any definite answers.

I am in a coffee shop eavesdropping on the conversation next to me. Across the street, some upholstered chairs sit out in the rain on an open porch. *Their* decompensation is imminent. The folks in the next booth are probably a good generation older than me.

"Remember the things our parents let us do back in the old days?" The slightly quavering voice of a man drifts over.

"Oh, nowadays kids are so overprotected. Remember the playground equipment then? Metal, with bolts, hard asphalt!" They all laugh out loud.

"I remember being on the swing and being pushed until it went all the way over. It was beautiful."

Another man chimes in, "I rode my bike around like a fiend, cutting in and out of traffic. Who ever heard of helmets?"

I yearn to go sit with them and drink my coffee. I want to be in their world, without protection, where broken legs and arms are just part of the game. Things heal, and you continue with your life. *They* weren't afraid all the time. They had definite answers.

A woman's voice: "I used to hop on and off of the trains." A moment of hushed respect.

"You did?"

"Oh, yes, all the time. It was the exhilaration of risk. I couldn't get enough."

"But how did you go from the boxcar out?" one of the men asks.

"Jump!" she exclaims. "Just jump and roll. It is the opposite sensation for you, the jumper. The train is still, and you are moving."

I go to the counter and pay. As I walk back past them, the man in a cap says, " . . . and powdered milk! Remember that? It was good enough for us."

I hear a muffled "Forever Young" from the depths of my handbag. "Yeah, Nick?"

"Hi, Mama," he says. He hasn't called me Mama in a long time. His voice is balanced. "I've been thinking. I don't want to just live alone in this apartment forever. I mean, I'm thirty-one years old now. I have to do something with my life. I think I need to save some money. Get a job."

When a boy is in his late teens, there is a synaptic pruning of sorts that occurs in the brain in order to mature and function in its adult form. It's a dispensing of the connective material that has built up since birth but is no longer needed, and it is quickly replaced. But there is a brief period of vacancy, when the brain is vulnerable to any sort of disruption. The mind is somewhat unprotected, and that is the stage of life when disease can make its appearance.

I have been told that there are eighty-six billion neurons in the brain. That is an unimaginable number. Virtually anything could happen. I have no idea what the final brew will be, but right now, something is percolating in my son's mind.

There is movement.

ACKNOWLEDGMENTS

Writing this book was a transmigration, and my gratitude goes to many people in my life.

To Craig, for always telling me that I was a writer, and then, one winter morning in 2017, telling me just go in my room and write the book already. Your belief in me was everything.

To my beloved squad, who read and listened and read and listened: Brooke Adams, Judy Landau, Carolyn Brooks, and Lynne Adams. You women are my ballast against the storm.

Thank you to my Larchmont Village women who delivered epic love and friendship: Jill, Stacy, Valerie, Madden, Gill, Jean, Judy, Melanie, Bebe, Carolyn, Kari, Mary, Dolores, Libby, Laura, Theresa, Bridget, Brenda, and Robin.

Thank you to Julie and Chris, who first took it seriously and then actually sat at a table with me for weeks and read the whole damn thing out loud. And cried.

Oh, and Samantha Dunn, who took it all apart, gave me back the pieces, and told me to now go turn it into a book. Then, on a street corner in Orange, California, she told me that she would never forget Nick O'Rourke, which was exactly what I needed to go on.

Thank you to the sublime Josie Adams for editing, insight, and clarity, and for always loving Nick.

To Shannon Hughes, for delivering the title to me.

All the gratitude to my sister who, as always, was there for me. Through the actual story and through the writing of the story.

My hand to my heart for Dr. Rod Amiri, who did, indeed, save us.

Thank you to the friends who are writers: Janet Fitch, whose generosity and support helped get this off the ground. Garth Stein for much-needed advice and reality checks. Elyn Saks for hope and inspiration, before and after I knew her.

Lavina and Sandy, I could not live without you.

My agent Deborah, who kept me on her desk against all odds.

The wonderful people at Turner Publishing, who showed me that all the cautionary tales had been wrong.

My beloved writing group at Corporeal, Writing in Portland: Daniel, Elyse, Liz, Michelle F, Michelle B, Kelsey, Gina, Sheila, and Rhea. What a privilege to sit at the table with you.

Forever love to Lidia Yuknavitch, who rearranged my DNA (as she would put it) with *The Small Backs of Children* on one lonely plane ride and then miraculously became my friend and teacher.

Thank you to my brother, who is my anchor.

Boundless adoration and gratitude to my three muses: Scarlett, Lucy, and Rose.

Thank you to the caregivers who, with impossible compassion and the mystifying ability to love all humans, changed everything and brought such goodness into our lives.

A bottomless gratitude to the quiet deliverers of divine intervention who rescue us again and again. The lady who folds the towels at Kaiser, the woman behind the cash register at Pollo Loco, you beautiful creatures who offer salvation to strangers in the form of a smile or a kind word and then go on your way. You are not forgotten.

Finally, and always, I am grateful for Nick, whose intrinsic goodness could not be diminished and whose gentle soul *is* perfect.